NO
TIME
FOR
NONSENSE

NO
TIME
FOR
NONSENSE

Self-Help for the Seriously Ill

by Ronna Fay Jevne, Ph.D. & Alexander Levitan, M.D.

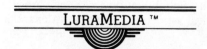
LuraMedia ™

© Copyright 1989 LuraMedia
San Diego, California
International Copyright Secured
Publisher's Catalog Number LM-613
Printed and Bound in the United States of America

Cover design and illustration by Carol Jeanotilla, Denver, Colorado.

LuraMedia
7060 Miramar Road, Suite 104
San Diego, CA 92121

Library of Congress Cataloging-in-Publication Data

Jevne, Ronna Fay.
    No time for nonsense.

    Bibliograpy: p.
    1. Chronically ill—Rehabilitation. 2. Self-care, Health. 3. Chronic
diseases—Psychological aspects. I. Levitan, Alexander. II. Title.
RC108.J48   1989   155.9′16   88-37250
ISBN 0-931055-63-6

Copyright Acknowledgments

Acknowledgments

We would like to acknowledge the following people who were so helpful with the book: our spouses, for their continuous emotional and practical support; Marion and Maurice Cardinal, for the use of their home as our creative headquarters; Bob Bajwa, Marianne Bibby, and Gary Grams, for their help in computerland. A special thank you to Marcia Broucek, our editor.

Contents

SECTION 1

INTRODUCTION

It's Time to Rock the Boat

Sorry. . .
The Rules Have Changed

Playing When the Odds Aren't Even

Why did we decide to write this book? We had to! Both of us have been working with, and for, seriously ill patients for over twenty years. Our experiences are primarily with cancer patients but please don't hold that against us. There will be no additional fee for the book if you have a disease other than cancer. Each of us has also had serious illnesses in the past that were associated with pain, anger, frustration, and eventual resolution — notice that we didn't say cure.

One thing we have learned is that seriously ill people don't have the time, patience, or stamina to engage in an extensive search for help with the multitude of problems which they may encounter.

We wrote this book to serve as a self-help manual for just such people. Think of it as a cookbook of recipes which we and others have found helpful in the past. We have kept the chapters brief and upbeat, not even attempting to cover all the literature that relates to the topics we are addressing. (We deliberately have chosen not to marinate you in academia. However, at the end of the book we have included some suggested readings that we feel are helpful.)

We want to make a difference in your life and in your illness. We have been fortunate enough to know many remarkable people who were able to improve dramatically both their lives and the outcome of their illnesses. We would like to share some of their techniques with you.

There are times when we'll use "we" and times when we'll use "I." (Grammar was never our strong suit.) Some of the chapters we wrote together; some we wrote individually. We hope this doesn't confuse you. See if you can figure out who wrote what.

Each chapter is brief because you don't have any time to waste. If a chapter doesn't appeal to you, skip it. Some of you will not be able to read a whole chapter all at once. And the last two chapters you're not supposed to read at all: One is for your family and close friends, and the other is for the professionals helping to care for you.

Our basic plan is simple. We'll tell you what you need to do if this book is going to make a difference in your life. We'll talk about the most common problems that people with a chronic or life-threatening illness run into, including physical, emotional, and practical difficulties. We'll give you our ideas about the skills and attitudes that we have seen patients use that have promoted their sense of health and well-being.

There are many books on the market that will tell you how to heal yourself; there are many more that will tell you how to die with dignity. We are interested in helping you learn how to live with your illness. (If you also manage to cure it, so much the better!) You already have the tools, skills, and equipment you need. Your body has some amazing built-in abilities. For example, you do not have to consult a reference book to heal a cut. Your body already knows how to do that.

Some people think they shouldn't try to cure illness with their minds. They'll take all kinds of bad tasting medicines, but they would never dream of rocking the boat. SORRY. . .THE RULES HAVE CHANGED! Rock away! It helps; we've seen it work. (For those of you who don't want to take our word for it, please see the references at the end of the book. They deal with the mind-body interaction, psychoneuroimmunology, and self-healing.)

For those of you who'd like to see for yourselves how much influence your mind has over your body, here's a simple exercise to try. Sit forward in your chair or stand up. Hunch your shoulders forward and put your chin on your chest. How do you feel? Depressed? Tense? Now, throw your shoulders back; hold your chin up high; take in a deep breath. How do you feel now? You have just helped your body to heal itself!

The same thing happens when you laugh — even more so! Every time you laugh, or even smile, you feel a little better. Therefore, throughout the book we've added the opportunity to laugh. . .at no extra charge, with no obligations.

Speaking of laughing, did you hear about the fellow

whose wife was concerned about him following his major surgery?

When she visited him the next morning, she asked him what kind of night he had had.

He thought he was making perfect sense when he replied, "No problem. It was great. I even managed to take a little walk on my own. And do you know what? When I went to the bathroom, God turned the light on for me."

The wife, concerned, consulted with the nurse in charge. "My husband said a really strange thing to me just now."

"Really? What was that?" asked the nurse.

"He said that when he went to the bathroom last night, God turned on the light for him," replied the wife.

At that point the nurse jumped up and ran down the hall, crying, "Oh, no, not the refrigerator again!"

If you had a hearty laugh, you are an excellent candidate for the techniques in this book. If you smirked and then checked to see if anyone was looking, you'll do fine. Just don't tell anyone you're into this stuff. If you frowned, you most likely *need* this book. Keep it under your mattress and sneak peeks into it late at night.

We hope to turn on some lights for you, but stay away from our refrigerator!

Because you are diagnosed as ill, it is not a requirement that you feel sick!

Ronna Fay Jevne

New Rules:
Your Part/Our Part

Who's Expected To Do What?

If you are going to get well and/or stay well, you are going to need a new set of rules. Perhaps one of your old rules is, "No play until the work is done," or "Father knows best." We're going to be making a number of suggestions for new rules but, ultimately, you'll be deciding which of the old rules to discard and what the new ones will be. Before we start working with you, we would like an agreement about what's our part and what's yours.

You can't even get your car fixed these days without a signed agreement. It's called a "work order." The nice thing with your car is that you just sign the work order and someone else does the repair. But when it comes to the repair of your body, we just teach you how to use tools you already have. But...you have to do the work. Before you start to work, though, we ask you to make a contract with us about how you will use your tool kit. We have some expectations of you...and of ourselves.

Other people have expectations of you, too. Unfortunately, many people will expect you to be a patient, and all that being a patient implies — usually, that you have less and less control over your own life. Medical people will tell you where to be and when to be there. If you are lucky, you will also be informed of why. Family and friends will tell you how you should feel and why they need you to feel differently. Some of them may expect everything to continue normally, and others will expect that somehow life is now totally different. Some friends will pick out condolence cards, while others start a fund for you to get to Mexico. Others with the "Coach Approach" will urge you toward herbal tea and long distance running. Some will expect you to "talk illness" all the time.

Invitations to meet other people's expectations will always be there. It is important to recognize these expectations for what they are and to decide which ones you will meet.

We have some expectations of you too. We expect that you are interested in feeling well, AND that you will doubt yourself on occasion. We expect you to:

- *Challenge your doubts, rather than abandon your efforts.*
  We understand that some days you'll be more hopeful than others. Having a few days where things don't go well makes it tempting to abandon hope. Notice what generates those doubts and choose to confront them, rather than let them undermine your commitment.

- *Pace yourself in reading this book.*
  It makes no sense to exhaust yourself reading about wellness. Consider yourself "in training" for wellness. If you were going to get physically fit, you wouldn't try the marathon the first day. You would begin with the exercise your body could handle. In much the same way, it is important to pace when and how you will work toward wellness.

- *Apply the suggestions in this book to YOURSELF.*
  YOU are the only one responsible for change in your life. Sure, it would be nice if the rest of the world were perfect, but it is important to start with what you have control over — that's you.

- *Take time to practice the attitudes and skills suggested.*
  This is a world of quickie cures and instant everything. Acquiring and sustaining well-being is not an overnight task.

- *Seek professional help for symptoms, physical or emotional, as necessary.*
  We will give you some help with this. Thoughts about when professional help is helpful or necessary will be discussed later.

The contract is two-way. We expect something from ourselves too. We plan to:

- challenge your commitment to your health;

- provide thought-provoking questions about your situation;

- introduce you to a variety of strategies for making a difference in your life;

- encourage your loved ones and your healthcare team to help you.

You may or may not like our style, but our goal is not necessarily to endear ourselves to you. We intend to say what we see and to tell what we know. Because we have been privileged to learn much from many people who have shared with us their journeys to health and to well-being, we agree not to fudge on the tough questions.

Life is the only game where the object of the game is to learn the new rules.

Ashleigh Brilliant

© Ashleigh Brilliant,
Santa Barbara, California

Locked on Target

Are You Ready for Commitment?

You may not like the word commitment.

After all, cousin Ted got "committed," and they have never let him out!

Every new government is committed to helping you, and you end up paying more taxes.

You may have said, "I do," and committed yourself to a marriage you wish you weren't in.

There is a good reason why marriage ceremonies do not let you say, "Well, maybe." Sometimes the only thing that gets us through tough spots in relationships — whether they be intimate partnerships, parent-child relationships, or friendships — is commitment. The same goes for getting something accomplished: Commitment is what gets you through the sluggish days of even the most creative project. It's no different when you're dealing with an illness. It's not wrong to feel like throwing in the towel, but it sure helps your staying power if you are committed.

Being committed to something is not a major triumph in itself. Lots of people stay committed to things that are unhealthy for them — physically and emotionally. They stay in jobs and relationships that have long since lost even the remote possibility of being good for them. They may say they are staying because they are "committed" — but that's not the word we would use! Does it make sense to be committed to someone or something which, after considerable time and effort, still obviously is going to kill you, or at least kill your spirit? Sounds more like fear to us.

Commitment means staying on target, remaining dedicated to what you set out to do. Commitment gets you where you want to go. But no one ever said that because you are committed to something, it would be easy. Matter of fact, it might be harder. The rewards are great, however.

It is highly unlikely that other people will ask you directly, "How committed are you to getting well?" Everyone will assume that you are! But there are all kinds of reasons why a person lacks commitment, and why illness, as long as it is not too threatening, is tolerated. Illness can:

- provide an excuse for not being as successful as you had dreamed you would be;

- provide the permission you need for taking care of yourself;

- get someone off your back;

- get you some caring from people who are otherwise insensitive;

- provide an income of some kind that you might not otherwise have;

- give you something to talk about if you don't have anything else interesting in your life;

- be, in your mind, a sign to the world that you were a hard worker;

- be a way of avoiding saying you are just too tired to face life;

- postpone some unpleasant decisions you are contemplating;

- be something you think is the doctor's responsibility to cure.

If you don't like looking at this list of possibilities, you might want to ask yourself, "Why would any of these bother me?" If you can clearly say that none of these applies to you, GREAT. Step one to being committed to your health is already accomplished: that is, you have no reason, however small, why you would prefer illness to wellness.

If one or more of these possibilities has a grain of truth in it for you, you are not alone.

The beginnings of our attitudes toward illness start in childhood. Illness is often a time when we are indulged, removed from the responsibility of school, excused from our chores, and awarded special privileges. We may have even received special gifts from people who care. That's all great, but there is the possibility that we learn that illness is somewhere to which we can retreat if we need some pampering, or if we wish to avoid something. As adults, there are other healthier ways of meeting our needs and discharging ourselves from obligations we do not want.

Think about it for a moment. If you are unhappy at work or in your present relationship, wouldn't resigning or separating make more sense than being sick? Ask yourself: "If I don't do something about the situation, how will my health be in three years?"

You might find, like Howard, that people are actually much more supportive than you expect they will be. Howard stayed in a marriage for a decade after he was sure it was emotionally over. He thought he was staying for the kids. When he suffered a major heart attack, he decided this was his ticket to change his stressful life. The response of his daughter to his decision was a supportive sigh of relief: "Well, Dad, it's about time!"

Even better than having no reason to be ill is to have a reason you want to get well and stay well. There are numerous studies that show that those individuals with a reason for living, despite chronic illness, live far longer than those without. The reason doesn't have to be profound. It can range from taking care of a pet to completing a life's work. It can be something specific in the future, such as wanting to see your daughter graduate. Then how about looking forward to seeing her established in adult life? Many a patient has remained alive to acquire the status of grandparent. If you don't like your children, stay around and spend their inheritance!

Or you may want to accomplish something specific: "I am not going to die until I have learned to play Beethoven's Fifth Piano Concerto"; or, "I will not die until I have knit sweaters for all of my nieces and nephews." (It helps if you have eleven siblings!)

What are your reasons for living? How about sharing the fall colors with someone you really care for? How about a starry sky, a rainbow, or a child's smile? Besides, if you die, who is going to look after your spouse or your dog? Who is going to teach your grandchildren about family traditions and the old country? Who is going to finish planning the conference program? How are you going to learn your new hobby?

Revenge worked for one man. He had been awaiting a settlement for injuries sustained in a car accident. The case lingered on and on. Finally, with a life expectancy of three weeks, he accepted a settlement that was to pay him so much per month until his death. He lived three years with a grin on his face.

You may be happy with your work, your partner, your social life, your situation in life in general. Great! That gives you an edge. You have built-in support and motivation to get well. But that is only part of what commitment is about.

The second aspect to commitment is to accept that the responsibility for contributing to your health, and ultimately for running your life, is *yours*.

A lung specialist we know decided to make it clear to patients that they share the responsibility for getting well. He refuses to see any patient who refuses to stop smoking!

It is not uncommon for patients to make someone else responsible for some, or all, of their care. It can happen without even consciously thinking about it. If you are a mother, you know this happens all the time. How many times does someone yell, "Where are my socks?" as if you were the sockkeeper of the world! With illness, all kinds of similar assumptions get built in.

Frank assumed because his partner did the cooking, she was also responsible for his weight. When Frank lost forty pounds everyone was concerned. His partner was feeling very badly that she couldn't get his weight up. She was even using the hospital's new cookbook which had high-caloric recipes for just such purposes, but Frank didn't like many of them. Both were quite startled when asked, "How did Wendy become responsible for your weight?" Wendy caught on quickly. She decided she would make the most pleasant high-caloric meals she could, but only Frank could eat them. She stopped feeling inadequate. Frank got the message, started eating, and gained weight.

What is it that you need to be committed to? Only what *you* want to be committed to! It is important to recognize that you limit your well-being to the degree that you limit your commitment. If you don't invest, you don't get the interest!

You need to decide what you will commit to. Consider these ideas and questions:

- The ultimate commitment is to run your own life. What parts of your life are you running now? Your financial life? Your emotional life? Your time? Your energy? Your decisions? If you aren't running them, who is?

- How committed are you to doing whatever is necessary to get well, or to managing your illness? How are you limiting yourself? Think about your answer. If someone you loved was the patient, would you like it if they gave the same answer?

- If getting well meant giving up some things, material or emotional, for a while, would you do it? For example, if it meant you had to sell the second car, would you do it? If it was your son who was ill, would it be easier to sell the car? How about if it meant a smaller house? How about accepting social assistance? What limits have you placed on your commitment?

- What about the emotional side of your life? Are you willing to give up controlling so much? (If you're asking, "Like what?", how would anyone else know? It's your life! Only *you* know what it is that you need to take more or less control of!)

- How long will you take to forgive yourself for your poor financial investment? What will you do with your guilt? How much of your life will you give to fear? How much of this do you think you have to do alone?

- How willing are you to learn new things? New attitudes? New skills? Think of an illness as winning a ticket to a place where you have to learn a new language and learn to do things you have never done before. (That's a lot to ask, isn't it?) Some people will spend a whole winter taking night classes just to learn the language of a country they want to visit. Yet, when they are ill, they don't read a single article on their disease. Puzzling, isn't it?

> ● On a scale of one to ten, how committed would you say you are to getting well? If we asked one of your close friends the same question about you, what would they say? Would there be any differences in your answers, and if so, how do you account for them?

It is never too late to learn commitment and to learn to use it to your advantage. Many people have avoided commitment. If you are one of them, you may be wondering if you have what it takes. Try it. It's like a muscle. Exercise it and it grows stronger. We'll help. Others will, too, if you ask. For you, learning commitment may mean going back to school to learn the basics of setting and meeting goals, becoming more assertive, dealing with your feelings.

Some of you may be saying to yourself, "I have spent my whole life being obliged or committed to this or that — the kids, the job, the whatever." Well, it's time to see if you are as good at being committed to self-care as you have been to being supermom or a workaholic. It may not be as easy as you think. You may have to undo some attitudes and behaviors. YOU have to be the focus of your commitment.

Commitment is the hardest step toward wellness, but commitment makes it easier to make good decisions about your health. It is like having an emotional budget that allows you to plan what you are willing to spend time, energy, and resources on. Of course, there will be unexpected expenditures, but they can be accommodated if you have good emotional credit or some savings.

Watch for that nonsense that suggests someone is actually sharing the illness experiences with you. There is a patronizing tone that goes, "And how are WE today, and how did WE like our breakfast, and are WE going for treatment soon?" "WE" can care. "WE" can help, but "WE" do not have the illness. YOU do. YOU have to do the getting well. YOU have to be the one who is committed. If you test "their" commitment, you may find "they" are not as committed as their "we" implies.

An elderly gentleman just a few days from his death decided to check out what "we" meant. He was just about to be helped back into bed, when he heard the words, "Let's get back into bed now, dearie." His eyes twinkled and he replied, "You first, my dear."

Just a word of caution. A problem sometimes arises when you are committed to your own health. Others may have something else in mind. For example, there are doctors who relish the god-like illusion of being totally responsible. We suggest you get yourself another doctor, or that you understand your doctor's limits and get on with your life. Your doctor may not be the one you want to discuss your relaxation training with (although he or she probably needs it!).

Some family or friends may suddenly decide that, since part of your body is not well, you have lost the ability to make even the simplest choices in your life. Without consulting you, they begin to make numerous decisions which you would like to continue to make. Sit them down, tell them you are dedicated in your efforts to getting well and are perfectly capable of making decisions. At the same time, thank them for their care. You may be amazed; they will probably be relieved.

Other people in your life may now need to learn to do for themselves what you have been doing for them all along.

In both cases, your friends and family will need a little training. This is new to them, too.

Yes, you could be labeled "difficult"! Would you rather be sick?

Don't be surprised that if you don't agree with someone about being depressed, anxious, or difficult, someone may order a visit from the psychologist (or social worker or psychiatrist). Let them come; and tell them the straight goods. Sometimes if the staff, family, or friends hear it from another source — particularly if the source has a few letters after his or her name — somehow they accept it. If you clearly show that you are motivated and responsible, it won't be long before people are on your team.

Being committed to your own well-being means being clear about what you want, about how you want to spend your time and energy; it means being willing to use the available resources.

This last point is important. There are no purple hearts given in this business. USE the resources that are available. You wouldn't remodel a house or fix a car without consulting advisors, gathering information, or using tools. Why try to do it with your body? Unfortunately, many of us take better care of our vehicles that we do of ourselves.

It can help to have reminders of your commitment hanging around. Put up some posters or signs where you can see them regularly. They *do* help. Here are some possibilities:

- Today I will make decisions for health.

- I am committed to getting well.

- Yes I CAN and yes I WILL!

- I care about getting well.

- I will have a nice day unless I've made other plans.

This attitude of commitment can be extended to the issue of your death, too. We have seen people suffer for a lengthy period of time because their relatives or friends could not handle their dying. Commitment includes having the right to decide when the fight is over. Some people may sense that, just as there was a time when they were ready to crawl, to walk, to go to school, to have their first job, it now feels natural to die. You have a right to acknowledge that you are ready.

Start exercising your commitment today. How willing are you to read this book? That would be a good first step on the road to wellness.

It is part of the cure to wish to be cured.

Lucius Annaeus Seneca (c. 4 B.C.–65 A.D.)

SECTION 2

PERSPECTIVE

How Bad Is It?

Disarming the Alarming

Let's Talk Stress

Stress is the catchword of the eighties! It is the topic of talk shows, pop psychology books, and sermons. Dinner parties are no exception. Conversations sound like a game show with the prize going to the person who has the most hassles. Stress is the explanation for your fatigue, your untidy garage, your short temper, and why your boss doesn't promote you. HARRIED and HURRIED, or WEARY and WORRIED, is the style of the day. It is almost trendy. How many times a week do you hear the words, "This is crazy — I am going to slow down"? Well, now may be the time, particularly if you have recently:

- put hairspray on your underarms;

- put your purse, instead of your letters, in the mail slot;

- arrived on time for a meeting, but on the wrong day;

- gotten to the grocery check-out and discovered you have someone else's cart;

- forgotten your phone number;

- measured where a nail goes, and then hammered it in the wrong place anyway;

- locked your keys in your car, only to have the locksmith point out that the passenger side was open all along;

- tried to find a friend's number in the phone book by looking under his or her first name;

- turned off the freeway at the exit that takes you to work—only it's Sunday!

Some stress is not so amusing. Have you ever:

- yelled at someone you care about?

- wanted to pack your stuff and leave because you couldn't handle it?

- gotten in a car accident and not even remembered where it was that you were going at the time?

- binged on booze, food, buying sprees, or work in order not to face something?

- cried totally unexpectedly?

- woken up anxious, night after night, not even sure about what?

- known you were not doing a good job of your work but felt like you just couldn't give any more to it?

Stress may be a trendy word, but it is a real experience with real consequences. Stress is what we experience when something is challenging, demanding, or threatening. The stress reaction system was originally designed to help our early ancestors survive in the natural world. If a tiger jumped out, the alarm system went off, and the body readied for action by preparing to flee or fight. Maybe there were a few optimists back then who said, "Here, kitty, kitty," but for most people, the pulse increased, the muscles tensed, the breathing changed, and the adrenalin started pumping.

We do not have tigers in our lives any more, but our bodies continue to set off the alarm system with any recognition of threat — physical or emotional. The stress reaction helps alert us to possible dangers and gives us extra energy to deal with them. It also helps us survive situations that call for fast action — like dodging an oncoming car. The feeling that goes through your body as someone else runs a red light and is coming toward you is definitely a stress response.

A stressor can be anything that is a source of challenge, demand, or threat. Response to the stressor varies with the situation and with each individual. The point is, the stress still happens. Ordinary life exposes us to stressors every day: driving to work, standing in line, raising kids, and holding onto a job are just the beginning of a long list of what can challenge us in an ordinary day.

There is nothing like having a fender bender on the way to work, then getting there late to find out that is the *one* day of the month the boss wanted to see you right away. Or sitting in the cafeteria next to someone who is telling you how great the ice cream is while you are having a salad because you are on a diet. Or deciding to forego your dental appointment in order to get your son to soccer, only to arrive home to find out that he has chosen this day to decide that soccer is "dumb" (in the meantime, he has created a full-fledged picnic in the rec room because he resents having to clean up, while his sister didn't remember to walk the dog!). . .and it is your night to make supper!

Granted, none of these things is shattering, but when they happen, you *do* feel stressed. If your reaction to stress is to tell yourself, "I am inadequate. I can't seem to handle the simplest things," you will feel vulnerable and inadequate. If you think, "Nothing ever goes right. Lousy drivers. Lousy kids. Who needs this?" you will feel angry and imposed upon. If you conclude, "Nobody helps. I have to do it all," you will feel burdened and tired.

There are healthier choices for dealing with stress. Keep reading. We will be talking about your choices throughout the book.

Remember: Good things are stressors, too. Surprise parties, family gatherings, promotions, going back to school — they all come with their challenges. The idea is not to be stress-free. The idea is to prevent, manage, or minimize the damage. The idea is to live life with the greatest degree of satisfaction.

Some people have the ability to make *everything* stressful. Some do it with poor decision-making: choosing what to wear, what movie to see, what gift to buy, or whether to have a face lift all become mini-crises. Others do it by believing they have to be involved in everything: their work, their community, their children's lives (even though their children are now grown adults living 3,000 miles away. . .probably with good reason!).

Our preoccupation with time is also a common culprit in creating stress. Some people drive as if it is important to get to the next stoplight *first*. They often do. Rarely do they think that they might also be the first to get a headstone.

This phenomenon of being in a hurry has infiltrated our society. Recently we observed a mom and dad who had brought all the kids grocery shopping. The parents were doling out eight items to each apparently cooperative youngster so that they could all go through the express line and make a quicker getaway.

We live in an age of fast foods, fast cures, fast cars, fast everything. It all takes its toll. What many people fail to recognize is that stress accumulates. Eventually, the body feels the wear and tear to which we expose it. The process is called aging. When the body is challenged beyond its limits, we become ill.

Stress is a known contributor to some illnesses. Note that we are not saying that stress *causes* illness; that is a scientific issue still being examined. But there are exciting studies investigating the body's response to different stressors. For example, there is a known link between stress and the immune system, and between the immune system and illness. That information is not new. Our grandmothers have been saying for years, "You will make yourself sick if you don't stop moping around." Friends have often given us the advice, "You better slow down or you're going to pay for it." But why some people pay for it and others do not is still somewhat of a puzzle. And so is the fact that we all behave as if we are going to belong to the group of people who escape the consequences.

If you feel that you have contributed to your illness by your choices in lifestyle, it is important that you spend very little time feeling guilty. (Perhaps you could spend a moment or two — it impresses your family and physician!) But then get on with dealing with your choices. At least you have things you can change!

Whether or not stress is a factor in the cause of your illness, what you are likely already recognizing is that illness brings its own set of stressors. With illness comes new concerns and challenges as your life changes.

There are investigations, and investigations, and investigations! Some are intrusive and unpleasant, if not downright embarrassing. A total stranger will probably ask you if your bowels have moved. If you have always been well, you won't know whether to be offended (after all, where could they have gone!) or afraid.

There may be pain. We have not met a single person who would rather be in pain than be comfortable.

Your body may change. It may not work the way it used to. It may even change shape or size.

Treatments can be the pits. The only thing worse is to hear that there is no treatment.

There is change after change. Your family and friends change, sometimes in ways you don't like. Your partner may start treating you differently or the kids may get out of control. Even if they are all super about the adjustments, you have the opportunity to feel like a burden. Your work is disrupted. Your social life changes.

For the first few weeks, there may be so many flowers in the living room, it looks like a funeral parlor. Then, suddenly, you wonder if people think you died. The telephone calls dwindle off. The get-well cards stop arriving. The visits stop. This is not uncommon. People go back to their stressed lives. They don't intentionally abandon you. And, of course, you may be bone-tired.

All these changes generate feelings: anger, fear, discouragement, frustration, guilt, and loneliness. To top it off, you may have difficulty discussing some of the feelings and changes with your family, friends, physician, or colleagues. Even if you want to, they may avoid the discussions. This is even more true if people think you are soon going to be a statistic.

Caregivers get stressed too. One veteran nurse attending a workshop on "Care of the Caregiver" was unsure if she had any stress. She didn't want to appear weak in front of her colleagues, so she inquired at the break as to whether waking in the night and finding herself going through the motions of adjusting an intravenous in the center of her living room would constitute being stressed!

Remember, stress varies from person to person and from situation to situation. We grow up in different families; we have different successes and failures, different fears, different skills, different resources; we believe different things about what life is and should be. So it is natural that we all have different amounts and types of stress in our lives when illness arrives.

Remember, too, that stress accumulates. Many of us behave as if we can just keep adding to our days. We add kids, mortgages, work, aging parents, coaching Little League, financial stress. At the same time, we withdraw energy, well-being, and satisfaction. Then we end up feeling bankrupt. It's like having a bank account and believing we can make withdrawals for years without making deposits. Illness is a time to start making deposits and thinking about where to invest the interest payments.

Having an illness provides you with an opportunity to re-think the way you live, to decide to continue those things which contribute to your well-being, and to abandon those which do not. At no other time will people give you as much permission, or put up as little resistance to the changes you may want to make, as they will now. Go for it. The life you save may be your own.

 If you ask me what is the single-most important key to longevity, I would have to say it is avoiding worry, stress, and tension. And if you didn't ask me, I'd still have to say it.

George Burns

First, the Biggies

Pain, Suffering, and Death

It is no fun being sick, but the worst part of the whole experience is imagining what might happen next. Well, in case you didn't know it, you're going to die! So are we all!

Death is part of life. Most of the cells in our bodies die and are reborn at regular intervals. Every living thing on this earth dies, almost as if that were part of the contract for being permitted to be born. Why should you or I be an exception? A deal is a deal, and we both have to die.

What most people are interested in is the *timing*. Sometimes death takes us more by surprise than we would like.

> A patient received a telephone call from her doctor who said, "I've got good news and bad news for you."
>
> "What's the good news?" asked the patient.
>
> "The good news is that you have twenty-four hours to live," said the doctor.
>
> "Wow! If that's the good news, what's the bad news?" inquired the patient.
>
> "The bad news is that I forgot to call you yesterday!"

In addition to timing, *compassionate care* from others is also of concern.

> A man came home from visiting his doctor and appeared very depressed to his wife. She asked, "What's wrong?"
>
> "The doctor said I have only twelve hours to live," replied the husband.

"What do you want to do about it?" asked his wife.

"First, I'd like to have you cook my favorite meal," said the husband.

"Yes, then what?" asked his wife.

"I want to go to bed and make love all night," answered the husband.

They had a wonderful meal and went to bed and made love repeatedly until they both fell asleep. The husband woke up at four a.m. and nudged his wife awake, saying, "Let's make love one more time. I don't want to sleep."

"Well, that's okay for you to say," replied his wife. "You don't have to get up in the morning."

As you can tell from this story, there is a limit to the amount of compassionate care any one person can give. But that doesn't have to be considered bad news. There is good news, too. Despite the fact that we are all going to die, this can usually be accomplished in a setting of dignity, comfort, love, and security, if you will follow a few simple rules. *The first rule is to define clearly the relationship between you and those who are caring for you.* Remember that the doctor, the nurses, and all the support personnel are your employees! You are paying them, and you have every right to define the kind of care that they give you.

Make sure that from the outset everyone understands who is calling the shots! Of course, you don't have a medical degree, but that doesn't mean that you can't decide what is best for you. When you hire a doctor, that doesn't mean you have to blindly accept everything suggested without question. It is important to establish from the outset that you reserve the right to call a halt to treatment if you deem it appropriate to do so, based on an informed and thoughtful decision.

The sequel to this fundamental tenet is *rule number two: You deserve an honest response to any question you pose about your illness and anything relating to it.* As is the case with most people caring for seriously ill patients, we have learned to respond as truthfully as possible to all patient inquiries. Telling the truth all the time makes life easier, too. There isn't the embarrassment of confusing those with whom you left out information and those with whom you were direct and honest.

Some well-meaning relatives and friends may request that certain facts, such as the diagnosis or prognosis, be withheld from patients. This even used to happen routinely when patients were being admitted to the National Cancer Institute or the Cross Cancer Hospital. Frequently we would hear the request, "Don't tell her what she's got." What nonsense! Even the most unenlightened patients realize that they are not being admitted to a cancer hospital for treatment of a head cold!

If you want to know more, or if you want to know *everything* about your illness, ASK FOR IT! You are entitled to this information, and you should have it if you wish. After all, who do you think gets the bill at the end, anyway?

Rule number three is that those caring for you must agree to abide by your decisions about your care, even if your opinion is at variance with theirs! If any member of the care team is uncomfortable with this, they have the right to withdraw from your care. But, as long as they remain on your team, their principal obligation is to keep you comfortable, informed, and secure in the knowledge that *your* wishes will be respected in regard to the type and extent of care you receive. This should apply even if your wishes are different from those of your loved ones or family.

Speaking about comfort, let's talk for a minute about pain. There are all kinds of modern ways to keep any patient comfortable under any circumstances. Some of the specifics will be discussed later in this book (see SECTION 6, page 153). Nevertheless, there is no reason why any patient with a serious illness should have to endure pain, unless that patient chooses to do so in order to attain a specific objective.

It is true that sometimes you have to choose between remaining fully alert and remaining comfortable. It may even be that you'll choose to stop treatment, even though that decision may hasten your death. That's your right to decide, as long as it is a properly-informed decision. If any member of the care team cannot abide by this rule, it's time to call in reserve players.

Let's talk about suffering. YOU MAY HAVE TO DIE, BUT NO ONE SAYS YOU HAVE TO SUFFER! Suffering is optional. You don't have to have it unless you choose to! Suffering comes from accepting someone else's expectations instead of your own. Suffering comes from being afraid to rattle the cage. Suffering comes from not expressing your feelings, including anger, fear, and even love. Especially love. Suffering comes from worrying about what tomorrow will bring instead of living today. Suffering comes from not availing yourself of the help that is there waiting for you.

Some of the suffering that comes with death and dying may come from artificially trying to delay death when it is imminent or from worrying about the experience before it happens. Surely you can find something more productive to worry about! How about whether you have told everyone you want to just how much you love them, and how nothing, not even death, can extinguish or reduce that love?

Now that we've mentioned it, let's talk a bit more about death. If people feared being born as much as they fear dying, there would be very few of us here! From what we have learned from people who have had a near-death experience, dying is not the anxiety-producing experience many of us fear. This is particularly true now that we can be assured of physical comfort during that process. That may sound as if it is easy to say — particularly since we haven't died.

We have, however, spoken with a lot of people who have been medically dead for an appreciable length of time, or who have visualized the death experience in a particularly vivid and convincing fashion. Almost without exception, they report a comfortable and beautiful experience from which they reluctantly returned to rejoin the living. They usually describe a sense of welcome, as if relatives or friends were waiting there to greet them, and a painless sensation of release from the physical limitations of their bodies.

Dying isn't something we can practice, so it isn't surprising that the unknown concerns us. In the face of death, all else begins to seem rather insignificant. But it is also in the face of death that we feel the most urgency to live. In the face of death, there is NO TIME FOR NONSENSE!

 Dying is part of living but only a small part.

Ashleigh Brilliant

Count Your Burdens

Getting Perspective on Your Problems

It was near Christmas of his tenth grade year when Troy and I met. He was referred to me to talk about his truancy. A small-framed kid with a wiry build and a contagious grin, he quickly admitted that, yes, he had missed a lot of school. He volunteered no information about his situation until I inquired further. Well, yes, he did have a few things he had been doing. His dad had died, leaving the family in considerable debt; his mom had no skills for employment, so he had opened a corner lot where he was making a killing selling Christmas trees; he had had to go out to the coast to help his sister who had gotten mixed up in drugs (and he was successful in helping her); and he was helping his other sister who was about to become a single parent. Other than that, he had no excuse. He was sorry if his absence had caused anyone any concern. He smiled, obviously unburdened by disclosing what would have been more than disconcerting to most of us and added, "Sometimes, you just have to do what you have to do."

I concurred, although I checked out his story to be sure I wasn't getting conned by a street superkid. It was all true. He had, however, left out his part-time job.

At his young age, Troy had developed several important attitudes and skills: He had figured out what needed attention first; he had put things in perspective; he had not blown anything out of proportion; and he had decided he was not powerless and had gotten on with his life. It was tough enough having so many challenges. He did not make it tougher by seeing them as burdens. He was not about to apologize for not being everything to everybody. He was just doing the best he could and preventing a difficult situation from becoming worse.

Feeling burdened is different from basic "whining." Whining is what we do when we don't intend to do anything about what is bothering us. Feeling burdened is what we do when we care about something and feel unable to influence it. In this chapter, we'll help you identify those concerns that are stressors for you, and, therefore, potential burdens. And, more importantly, in the next section we'll help you take note of the resources in your world to help you take charge of the challenges.

It helps if you know what you are up against.

Where is the sense of burden most likely to come from in your life? There are, after all, lots of possibilities. There are the daily practical hassles, the changes at home and at work, the "big" questions — the ones about meaning and questions of the "what-is-life?" variety. And then there are all the feelings.

You could defer to someone else to run the rest of your life. That is really no problem. Lots of people do it. Just be prepared to accept their mistakes. (And, be assured, they will make them!) That's because they are not you and, therefore, the best consultant has just abandoned ship. Taking charge of your life doesn't mean you personally take care of everything. It means you manage your life, you retain the right to make decisions about what affects you. Even if the options are not so great, you still run your life working with the circumstances in which you find yourself.

There is no magic way to do this. We suggest that now is a good time to start a notebook where you can see things on paper. You don't have to be so explicit that if someone was inconsiderate enough to pick it up, they would be disturbed by what they read. (On the other hand, what are they doing reading your notebook, anyway?) You could put a big note on the front:

CONFIDENTIAL — DO NOT READ

or

DON'T EVEN THINK ABOUT READING THIS

or

PUT THIS DOWN — CONTENTS ARE PRIVATE

or perhaps you prefer

SEX LIFE OF AN UNDERGROUND AGENT: CONFIDENTIAL — DO NOT READ

(Of course, if you use this title, they'll be sure to read it!)

If you section off your notebook, you can have sections for doctor's appointments, medications, medical tests and results, things to do, questions and problems, and a section for "my thoughts." (You may want to keep "my thoughts" in a separate journal.)

Some people use an "imaginary" notebook where they write notes to themselves, but the advantage of jotting your notes down is that, by getting them out of your head, you will have more room to think.

This chapter is much like the work order we described in the chapter on "New Rules." You are making out a work order for yourself. The more specific you can be, the more you will be able to sort out those things over which you do have control and those you can only influence with attitude. You need to be honest with yourself. Only you will know if you have been scrupulous.

Awareness and prioritizing of concerns is a first step toward coping. You don't have to know how to solve things at this point. Remember, there are no right or wrong answers. It's your *life* you are reviewing; it's not a driver's test you are trying to pass.

We've adapted a scale developed by Kanner, Coyne, Schaefer, and Lazarus, some research folks who are looking into the stress of everyday hassles. Their work points out that the little things can get us into trouble as often as the biggies. As you review the possible stressors suggested by the following stress inventory, sort them out into three lists, according to their intensity or priority in your life:

Major Stressors	Medium Stressors	Minor Stressors

As you create your lists, write yourself a little note about anything that you want to think about some more. Consider this as a kind of interview with yourself.

GETTING ACQUAINTED WITH MY BURDENS

Health and My Body

physical illness
medical treatment
side effects of treatment
pain
declining physical abilities
sexual problems or changes
relationship with my doctor
difficulties in seeing or hearing
difficulties in moving around
gaining or losing weight
changes in eating habits
no fresh air
trouble relaxing
no exercise
low energy
problems with my bladder or bowels
too much alcohol, drugs, or smoking
concern about how my body looks
others?

Financial Stressors

not enough money
no financial planning done
no one to manage the money
others?

Hassles with Work

lack of job security
problems with co-workers
dislike for work
hassles with supervisors
unchallenging work
difficulties with responsibilities at work
others?

Hassles with Other Things I Have to Do

car maintenance
transportation problems
child care
pet care
meal preparation
others?

Family Related Stressors

not enough time with my family
problems with
  – parents
  – children
  – spouse/partner
  – other relatives
household routine disrupted
others?

Difficulties with Handling Tasks and Problems

difficulties with redistributing my responsibilities at home
concern about not being able to do jobs I used to do
difficulties making decisions
feeling conflict over what to do
regrets over past decisions
a feeling of not doing things well
too many things to do
others?

Concerns for Friends and Relationships

problems with friends
friends and relatives are too far away
not seeing enough people
feeling lonely
prejudice or discrimination from others
conflict with others
inability to express myself
fear of being abandoned
don't know what to tell people about my illness
afraid to see old friends
others?

Concerns about Feelings

feeling angry
feeling afraid
feeling sad, crying
feeling depressed
feeling out of control
feeling guilty
feeling inadequate
feeling no one cares
feeling no one understands
feeling left out of things
others?

Concerns about Life and Meaning
troubling thoughts about the past
troubling thoughts about the future
unsure about how to plan for the future
why me?
why now?
thoughts about death
concern about the meaning of life
    – who am I?
    – where am I going?
    – what do I want from life?
    – what is a meaningful life?
    – is there any purpose to this whole thing?
others?

What did you discover? Take some *think time*. It's an old custom that people used to practice. They would sit and think. No radio. No television. Just sit. And think. Take a little piece of information and think about it. Ask yourself questions and listen to whatever comes up. Inside of you is an "Inner Guide." Listen to what your Guide has to tell you. If you get to know your Guide, you will have a very helpful resource throughout your illness.

Here are some questions that might help you get started:

- How does this compare with any other time of my life?

- If I had to rank order my stressors, which would be of most concern; which would be of least concern?

- If I could solve only three problems in the next week, which ones would they be?

- How did I decide these things are of concern?

- Am I making my illness better or worse by the way I think about it?

- Am I going to make these stressors burdens or challenges?

- Do I want to do anything differently about any of the stressors right now?

Getting perspective on your problems can help. You can see which ones are related to illness and which ones are just part of life. You have the possibility of preventing some and minimizing the damage of others. You may be able to control more than you first thought. Then, one last question. Ask yourself, "Do I need to UP MY ASSETS?"

 The higher the mountain, the greater the view.

Ronna Fay Jevne

No Time for Nonsense

A Time for Life Management

There's not much doubt that your life got complicated when you became ill. Ah! But it also got simpler. Now you do not have to apologize for missing the fundraising meeting or the golf tournament, and no one expects you to coach Little League this year. It can get even simpler. You can do less.

Granted, a few things got added to the list — like how to get to treatments, how to pay the mortgage, how to run a household with four hours of energy a day, and how to deal with scared friends.

You have to decide. This is a time that can overwhelm you or you can decide to manage the challenges. Not DO it all. MANAGE it. This can be a time unlike any other previous time in your life and unlike any time following your recovery. This is YOUR time.

Time is really no different. Only you can be. There are the same twenty-four hours in a day, the same seven days in a week. You can create difficulty for yourself if you keep the same expectations for yourself during this time as you have had for other times. By so doing, you can successfully drain yourself, worry your family, and take longer to achieve a sense of well-being.

What we are talking about is changing your priorities, and we know that isn't easy. Then again, lots of people have never had any priorities, let alone decided to change them. They just live day to day, thinking there will always be enough days.

Think about it. If someone made a movie of your life in an average week while you were well, what would they conclude about what is valuable in your life? Would you be one of those who said, "Oh, my family is important," and yet the video would show a series of meetings, shopping trips, and evenings in front of the TV? What would the video show about taking care of yourself? Regular sleep? Good meals? Healthy relationships?

Now that you are ill, there is less room for choices that are not what you intend. YOU come first. That's hard for most of us. Try it. Say, "I COUNT." First a little subvocal whisper. Now louder. Can you say it out loud? How about when the doctor comes in? It is time to realize that if you don't put yourself first for a while, there's not going to be a you. If you don't put yourself first, you are not giving recovery your best shot. Albert Schweitzer called it "benevolent egotism." He meant that when we really take good care of ourselves, in a total way, then we have something to offer others.

If you are well enough to keep up many of your activities, you still have to get to treatments. You will have to decide what you will exchange. You cannot just keep adding.

As for Aunt Alice, if you don't want to see her, this is a good time to put her at the bottom of the list. Setting priorities in terms of relationships is important. And it is not wrong. If you are unwilling to be around supportive people, and if you continue to be around people you really would like out of your life, the road to health will be traveled more slowly.

Mabel is a person with breast cancer who found out that her disease had spread to her lungs and bones. As well as taking her chemotherapy, she decided she would not worry about whether she was going to die, but that she would take charge of the time she had. She was tired of always being between her new husband and her sons. And she had always wanted to live on a farm with horses as a hobby. She decided to give up her anger and her sense of powerlessness. She moved to an acreage, bought the horses, and announced to her family that anyone who was interested in living in harmony was welcome. And she meant it. She is still riding five years later.

How about the day-to-day things? How important is it that the lawn is edged? Could just cutting it be enough this year? Do all the meals have to be banquets? How willing are you to have a "fend-for-yourself-night," or will you stay locked into believing you are the only one who can prepare a meal? If they do not know now, they should be learning. You could use the time for taking a bubble bath or listening to some music. Look around. Part of the problem is that you have not asked the question, "What am I doing that my children, my partner, or a friend could help with?" The real problem is not whether things *can* be done differently, but whether you are *willing* to have them done differently, willing to plan so that they happen differently, willing to treasure yourself and those you care about enough to set new priorities. This is NO TIME FOR NONSENSE!

Where are you going to start? Or are you hearing a little voice that's saying, "Well, this is all well and good, BUT. . ." But what? Are you going to influence your own life or not? Take a good look at the areas of your life affected by your illness and the resources you have for meeting new problems and challenges. It only makes sense that the person with the compass has the advantage in getting across the desert. Are you going to set a course or be blown about by circumstances? What's the old song, "I'm just a drifter"? Of course, you might prefer the lyrics of another song, "I did it my way." It's your choice.

If you decide to get on with things, here are a few questions to think about:

- How determined am I to get well?

- What decisions do I have to be considering?

- Whose help do I need?

- What might I need to learn. . .
    – to say "yes"; to say "no"?
    – to deal with feelings?
    – to communicate more effectively?

- How am I going to start?

We recommend that you start by "upping your assets!"

There is only NOW.

Ronna Fay Jevne

SECTION 3

RESOURCES

Up Your Assets

Up Your Assets

Taking Inventory of Your Resources

Two little boys, Tommy and Mark, were placed in a room full of horse manure and given a plastic sand shovel. Tommy, discouraged by the situation and appalled by the smell, cowered into one corner and began whimpering as he bemoaned his fate. Mark manned the shovel and began with gusto to move the manure.

Tommy, puzzled by the behavior, timidly inquired, "Why are you doing that?"

To which Mark replied, "Somewhere in here there has to be a pony!"

Was Tommy a wimp or was Mark wasting his time? Both were facing a difficulty. At least Mark's approach included hope. In facing the difficulties in life, some kind of hope is an important component. The more resources you feel you have, the more likely you will feel hopeful.

There is no point sitting in the corner hoping someone will rescue you. And there is no point bemoaning the resources that you *do not* have. Not everybody has everything or does everything well. There is no point wishing you were a gifted musician if your talent is growing petunias.

In our experience, we have seen that people have the potential to use what they have and to learn what they need to learn. Yes, if you are over fifty, we mean you, too. Yes, an old dog can learn new tricks. Don't forget, old dogs have more experience. The first hurdle to conquer is the idea that you have to be who you have always been, do what you have always done. If changing means surviving, we recommend a little change.

We think that the things you need to manage your illness and to get well fall into six categories. The next six chapters will deal with each of these categories in detail, but take a minute now to read through the brief synopsis provided here. Let your mind begin to think about what you *do* have going for you and where you have an opportunity to be more effective.

1) ACCURATE INFORMATION

Getting information is a first step to understanding and to making good use of your resources.

What information do you want? What information do you need? Sometimes there is a difference. How are you going to find out the facts? Who is the keeper of the secrets? What do you understand about your disease? Your treatment? Your rights? Hospital procedures? Available services?

2) A POSITIVE ATTITUDE

We hear all the time, "You are making yourself sick," or, "If you don't stop that, you are going to be ill." How often have you heard, "You can make yourself well"? If one is true, so must be the other. We all know or have heard of someone who has overcome some kind of insurmountable odds, whether it was illness or disadvantaged circumstances, and gone on to be a winner. Have you thought of being one of those people? Perhaps you already are. You are reading this book. How serious are you about developing an attitude that gives you every possible advantage? Can you think even now of attitudes that are self-defeating? Can you think of someone whom you can emulate in order to develop a positive attitude? Do you understand and believe the body and the mind are interconnected? Just think about when you are angry. How does your body feel? What could you be saying to yourself that would help?

3) A SENSE OF HUMOR

Think about someone you really like and feel close to. What are their three most important qualities? A good sense of humor is probably one of them.

People who can retain their sense of humor despite personal

tragedy are far more likely to survive than those who surrender to the circumstances. Humor is an emotional shock absorber; it enables us to get over the bumps without being jarred senseless. Even the most horrid circumstances can be improved by telling a joke or retaining a sense of humor. As a matter of fact, there are circumstances when humor can actually be life-saving. The Nazi death camps were a good example of this. Survival depended on being able to call upon a deep resolve to survive and to surmount present circumstances, and many inmates recall that humor was an important factor. One of the traditional Jewish curses illustrates this point: "May you have a hundred pearls, may you have five hundred rubies, may you have a thousand diamonds. . .all in your gallbladder."

4) PEOPLE WHO CARE

Ultimately, you are responsible for your own life, but it sure helps if someone will take in the mail while you are in the hospital. Things can be easier if you are able to arrange a little help in times of pressure. This is true emotionally as well as physically. Who is out there to help, and with what? Not every friend can help in the ways you might have expected.

Once you've gotten people to agree to help, what do you do with them? Making the best use of your support system takes some management. Without a little organization, you end up with six visitors on Tuesday and none the rest of the week; you have the home care nurse arriving for your long-awaited enema just as the minister has come with communion. Not good timing!

How do you get the most help with the least imposition? Can you ask for help? Can you handle it if someone has to say, "No"? Is everyone bringing flowers, but there is no one to take Cindy to music lessons? Is the freezer full of date squares but not a single casserole? What do you need to do to make more effective use of your support system?

5) YOUR OWN SKILLS

You have an endless list of skills that you probably don't even notice using each day. You cook things, fix things, organize things, decide things, move things, drive vehicles, phone people, order things, purchase things. You may have developed some specialized skills, too: taking photographs, motivating people, tuning the car engine, arranging flowers, carving, making pastry, fixing the lawnmower. Then there are the relationship skills: helping people feel wanted, making them laugh, encouraging them. Are there things that you can do that you hadn't thought of as skills? We often do not give ourselves credit for having developed skills or for using them.

By combining skills or using them in new ways, you may find creative ways to overcome obstacles put in your way by illness. An executive manager, for example, was delighted to find that, when he applied the same planning skills he used in business to the task of getting well, he came up with a six-month prospectus which outlined his wellness-recovering activities. Because he was a workaholic, he had the skill of discipline to stick with the plan.

There may be skills you don't have that you want to learn. Perhaps there are different ways that you would like to communicate or to handle your feelings. Are you able to drift off to sleep quickly and do you know how to take "one minute vacations"? Would you benefit by learning something about nutrition or about back care?

Are there skills you need to develop? In later chapters we will be talking about the importance of skills of assertiveness, handling feelings, and learning to relax.

6) INNER RESOURCES

The human spirit may be the richest resource we have. You can strengthen or deplete it by how you think, what you feel, with whom you associate, and by how you regenerate. Whether you express your spirituality through a traditional faith or through any number of other possible outlets, that special part of you that is uniquely you and yet somehow interwoven with the universe is a vital force for health. You don't have to be a Mother Teresa or an Albert Schweitzer. Being a dedicated parent or a conscientious employee may be your way. Loving music, dabbling in oils, or being a good neighbor are all ways of caring for and expressing your spirit. Notice who and what strengthens or diminishes your spirit; notice when your spirit seems vibrant and energetic. You can make choices toward joy and purpose.

Before reading any further, take a few minutes to check the condition of your resources. After you have read the following directions, close your eyes and allow yourself to picture this scene:

Imagine that you are walking along a most pleasant
valley with a wise and gentle person. You are carrying a

notebook with you and talking about the resources that
we've just described:
  – accurate information
  – a positive attitude
  – a sense of humor
  – people who care
  – your own skills
  – inner resources
Perhaps you find a pleasant place to sit where the view
is very refreshing or perhaps you walk side by side, as
old friends, intimate and yet separate. Take this time to
discuss with the wise person how well prepared you are
for a challenging journey that you know you are about
to embark upon. Talk about the resources which are
especially strong for you and the degree to which you
feel well-equipped. Listen for the advice of the wise
person as to which resources you need to strengthen
and how you might go about doing so. You can make
any notes you want in your imaginary notebook.
Perhaps you will want to have more than one discussion
with your wise person. He or she is available to you
whenever you are willing to quiet yourself and seek
guidance.

After you've completed this visualization, you may want to jot
down some of your thoughts in a "real" notebook. Let yourself begin
to imagine some ways you could increase your asset inventory.

  ● You could put a sign on your lawn declaring what you
    need.

  ● How about putting an advertisement in the newspaper?

  ● Call a couple of churches. See if they live up to their
    word.

  ● Ask for direction from your doctor.

  ● Every crisis line can tell you what resources are in town.

  ● Every reasonably-sized city has a volunteer center.

The next six chapters are devoted to discussing resources. Read the chapters in any order you want, but pay particular attention to those chapters that discuss areas where you need to UP YOUR ASSETS.

Never underestimate the nature of the problem; never underestimate your ability to meet it.

Adapted from Norman Cousins

Can You Spell What You've Got?

Getting Accurate Information

I can recall my first trip to Europe. I was preparing to travel from Frankfurt to Copenhagen by train. I had heard that it was customary for the occupants of train compartments to share food at mealtimes. I accordingly did some shopping before getting on the train and bought some bread and cheese to share with my future traveling companions. I was intrigued to note that, in Europe, Camembert cheese was sold in easy-opening metal cans, but I thought little of it.

Eventually the occupants of my train compartment began to take out various items of food and started to eat and share them. I did the same. The compartment was heated, as it was October at the time. Within seconds of my opening the can of what turned to be *aged* Camembert, people started looking at each other and asking, in German, "Where is that horrible smell coming from?" "From the American's rotten cheese!" was the response.

Eventually all the other occupants of the compartment gathered their belongings and stalked out, leaving me sitting in malodorous privacy. I really made friends and influenced people that day!

Coming into the world of illness is a little like traveling in a foreign country. It seems like everyone is speaking a foreign language and that everyone *except* you seems to know what they are doing and where they are going. Learning to get around in this new Land of Oz depends on your ability to figure out a few things.

In order to get the greatest assistance from those caring for you, it is necessary for you to understand as much as possible about your illness. You do not need to become a world expert, but you should understand what is known about the cause of your illness, its normal course, and the usual treatment.

There are various sources of information available to you. The first is your doctor. It is best to talk with doctors when they can take the time to answer all of your questions. During morning rounds, in the cafeteria, or in the hallways are not the best places if you want to feel good about your discussion. Ask, "When would be a good time to have a talk with you?"

Come to the meeting prepared with a list of questions that you want answered. Ask all the questions you wish, even those you think are "dumb!" There is no such thing as a dumb question where serious illness is concerned. Make sure that all of your questions are answered fully and completely.

- "Is the therapy proposed for me the best that I could receive anywhere? Are there alternative therapies available only elsewhere?"

- "Do you feel that there is any need for further consultation about either the diagnosis or the therapy? If not, why not? If so, with whom?"

- "Would it be possible for me to talk to another person with my kind of illness who has already received the therapy you propose for me?"

- "Are there any support group meetings for people with my kind of illness that would be helpful for me or my family to attend?"

- "Are there any national foundations or organizations established for helping persons with my type of illness?"

- "Is there anything else I should ask that I haven't asked yet?"

Sum up what you think your doctor has said before you leave, so your doctor has an opportunity to correct any misunderstandings. Bring a tape recorder or take notes so that you can recall your doctor's answers later. Be prepared for the fact that you will forget a good deal of what you are told. If possible, have someone close to you accompany you to the session. You can compare notes with that person later if questions arise as to exactly what was said.

It is especially essential that you be well-informed about medication. You need to wonder what those wonder drugs do. Keep a list of your medications in your wallet so that you always know the names and dosages. If you experience anything unusual after beginning a medication, inquire whether there is any relationship to the drug you have begun. It goes without saying that if you normally take three little red ones and one big yellow one, and you are delivered three yellow ones and a blue one, ASK, "Is there is a change in my medications?"

Patients are notorious for not following their medication regimes. This is usually the result of people not understanding what their medication does, how it does it, what it affects, and why it is important to take it as often and as long as prescribed. If you are lacking information or understanding, ASK, ASK, ASK. If you have to ask four times before you understand, that's fine. It is YOUR life. It is into YOUR body that the medication is going. Never share medication with others and never alter your own medication on the basis of a friend's advice. That is a decision for you and your doctor.

What about the other people in your life who want to know what's going on? There are some things that need to be settled with family and friends with regard to information. How much will everyone know? Are there going to be any conspiracies of silence? You need to define the terms under which communication should occur. For example, is the doctor free to discuss your illness with any other members of your family, and, if so, with whom? Let your doctor know with whom you would like to share matters. Ask your doctor when it would be convenient to schedule a family conference with all members of your care team so that family members can ask all the questions they wish. You might also want to consider if there is anyone who you would feel confident to speak for you, if you are weary.

How *much* people want to know varies from culture to culture and from family to family. In some cultures it is considered beneficial for the patient to know almost nothing. Other people simply *prefer* to have very little information. One elderly woman who had had breast cancer for twenty-six years and whose bone scan was being used for teaching purposes (because theoretically she could not have been walking around with so much bone disease) replied to an inquiry about how she felt by saying, "Well, this darn arthritis gets worse each year." She seemed quite capable of ignoring the many written reminders that indicated she was attending a cancer center. She had all the information she wanted. She needed her cane for her arthritis!

Some people feel very strongly that children should be protected from some information. Children are surprisingly observant, however, and often are aware of what is going on. Jason's parents made a decision to withhold from him until after Christmas that his dad had been diagnosed with terminal lung cancer. After the excitement of opening his gifts on Christmas morning, Jason turned to his parents and said, "I had a dream last night that Dad was going to die. Is Dad going to die?" Needless to say, they were caught off guard. Kids seem to have radar and suffer, not from difficult circumstances, but from the supposed protection of their parents. They have a need to be included. Our experience suggests that children have much less difficulty dealing with the straight goods than do adults. We recommend making an agreement that they can ask any question and you will give them what understanding of the answer you have. We believe in honesty with children. If you lie to them once, they may question if you would lie to them again. If things are not going to be okay, do not assure them things will be fine. Some things are going to change. They have a right to know.

The difficulty with information and who gets it arises when people feel they are lied to or left out, or that they are unduly burdened with information that someone else does not have. When and what do you tell friends? Do you tell your elderly grandmother who herself is ill? Do you keep attending church functions? If so, how do you handle all of the, "I was so sorry to hear," "You're looking so pale," "Is there anything we can do?", "My mother had something just like this" comments. At times like these, you have to decide whether to stretch the symptoms a little bit to include deafness!

Your Aunt Myrtle who was a nurse in the Crimean War is an unlikely source of current information about anti-inflammatory drugs for Crohn's disease, so you may not want to get into a lengthy discussion about it with her. You will get as much free advice as you can tolerate during an illness. Some of it may be useful and some is just plain dangerous!

Don't be disappointed if your doctor answers some of your questions with, "I don't know." Doctors don't know everything about everything! But they can direct you toward the latest information on any specific illness.

Some of these resources include the hospital and the hospital medical librarian. Most medical libraries can perform a computer search on any topic to find out about the latest developments relative to any illness. In the event that your hospital does not have this capability, this same search can be done 'in response to a mail request with a slightly longer turn-around time. The local medical society or regional medical school is a good resource as well.

Once a computerized literature search is available, ask to see it. If certain articles seem particularly pertinent, ask to obtain copies of these for your own and your doctor's reading. The same persons who did the literature search can help you obtain the articles. If you do not understand some of the terms used, ask to use a medical dictionary and ask the medical librarian to help as well! Take the time to analyze any data presented by going to the original sources and reading them, if at all possible. If you are intimidated by the idea of reading scientific information, find a friend who is not and ask your friend to translate.

There are a variety of self-help and support organizations available to help individuals who are seriously ill and their families, such as I Can Cope (U.S.), Share and Care (U.S.), and Cansurmount (U.S. and Canada). I Can Cope is designed to educate cancer patients and their families about cancer and its treatment; Share and Care is designed to provide emotional support for cancer patients and their families; Cansurmount is an organization of recovered cancer patients who visit newly diagnosed patients to give them the inside scoop on what to expect from their treatment and to answer any questions which patients may be reluctant to ask their doctors. Although these organizations are primarily for cancer patients and their families, similar support organizations exist for most other serious illnesses.[1]

Many of the chronic illnesses have national and international support organizations designed to foster research in the diagnosis and treatment of that particular disease. Among these are the Multiple Sclerosis, Diabetes, Arthritis, Sickle Cell Anemia, and Hemophilia foundations, to name a few. For AIDS patients, there are many organizations, including the National People with AIDS Coalition and the

---

[1]For further information regarding support organizations for people with serious illnesses, people in Canada can contact the Health Promotions Directorate, Health & Welfare, to get a list of health promotion agencies in Canada. People in the United States can contact their state Department of Health.

Canadian AIDS Society, as well as the National AIDS Hotline, 1-800-342-2437 (U.S.).

If for some reason there is no foundation for your particular disease, here's your chance: START ONE!

Illness is a word — not a sentence.

Ronna Fay Jevne

The Altitude of Your Attitude

Maintaining a Positive Attitude

If you have a good attitude, you are your own best resource. It has been said, "You are what you eat!" Feed yourself enough junk food, and you will feel sick. We have all done it. It has also been said (not so commonly) that, "You are what you think." The idea of the power of positive thinking has been around a long time. We have a variation on it: Don't think anything that is not really true for you.

For example, it is not effective to say, "I am feeling well," when you are nauseated and vomiting. It makes more sense to say to yourself, "I am looking forward to feeling better than I am at this moment. I believe I will feel better very soon." If you look in the mirror and see a body that they would use for a "Feed the Starving of the World" commercial, it is difficult to say, "I am beautiful. My body is a work of perfection." What you might be able to say is, "Thank you, body, for continuing to fight when you are so weak. I will help you in all the ways that I know how."

Your mind does not like junk food any better than your body does. Feed your mind the wrong thing and it wants to vomit, too. Discouragement and anxiety are fed by fearful thoughts. Hope and calmness are fed by thoughts of how to cope. Saying to yourself just before the fourteenth vial of blood is drawn, "This is going to be awful," is less helpful than saying, "I am glad I have something to look forward to this afternoon. This will be over in a few moments. I know it may be unpleasant, but I have handled unpleasant things before."

Many people are unaware of what they are thinking. By becoming more aware of your thoughts, you can control them much more readily. Practice now. Tell yourself something constructive. . .

What did you say to yourself? If you read the instructions and then passed on quickly to this paragraph, that's not enough. Your mind is like a computer. It was programmed years ago and needs an update in order to manage an illness. Learning to think constructively was likely not in the original program. Some of the original programming may have consisted of mottoes that you were told to live by. What are your mottoes? Recognize any of these?

- If you start something, finish it.
- Owe no one money and you'll have no problems.
- Never say no to opportunity.
- Get them before they get you.
- A stitch in time saves nine.
- Love your neighbor.

Do any of these mottoes still make sense for your situation? Some will, some won't.

Many of us did not grow up programmed with these kinds of thoughts:

- Take care of your body.
- Think good thoughts.
- Trust those who help you.
- There will be a better day tomorrow.
- Someone will help in a time of need.
- It's okay to need.

What you need is a program that works for this period of time in your life. Write down the new mottoes you will live by. Put them on a poster or in your journal and remind yourself of your new mindset.

You can actually improve your chances of well-being with a positive attitude. If you *think* you can be well, your body is more likely to respond to your belief. Yes, your body is like a personality: it feels, wants, dreads, enjoys — even believes and trusts.

(Here's an important note for you if you are facing surgery. There is evidence that the body hears under anesthesia. Tell your surgeon you want the operating team to say only constructive things about you during your operation, that you expect they will be a part of a team effort with you in helping your body believe in its capacity for healing.)

It is important to remember that your emotions play a large part in the way your body feels. When you're depressed, lonely, or afraid, things will bother you a great deal more than when you're in a more positive frame of mind.

Perhaps you have heard the song that was popular many years ago which was titled "Accentuate the Positive." If you don't remember it, the concept was to emphasize the positive, ignore the negative, and don't concern yourself with anything in between.

We all tend to have negative thoughts from time to time. So how can you manage to be continually in a positive state of mind, you might ask? The answer is: you can't! No one can be positive and upbeat for every moment of their existence. The idea is to do it as much as possible.

Instead of letting negative thoughts gain mastery over you, tell yourself, "These are just negative thoughts, and I really don't need to have them." Then think of something positive to take their place. In some cases it has been useful for patients to do something else whenever negative thoughts occur.

We all have a part of us that periodically needs to be reoriented to a more positive approach. This type of reorientation has been called "Ordeal Therapy" and is based on the idea that whenever we have a negative thought, if we do something which is good for us to do, but which we dislike doing, we will learn to stop having negative thoughts.

One patient, for example, who absolutely detested poetry forced herself to memorize four lines of poetry whenever she had a negative thought. She would carry around a book of poetry in her purse so that she would be continually prepared should negativity rear its ugly head. Not only did she stop having negative thoughts, but she eventually began to really like poetry and read it avidly.

Another patient found that her insomnia disappeared after three nights of making herself get up to do housework rather than allowing herself to stay in bed and worry. One woman, when pain woke her up at three in the morning, forced herself to shower and drive to work. Her actions told the pain in no uncertain terms that she would not tolerate any interference. If the pain insisted on being there, it could just expect to have to go to work with her!

Although this approach may sound, at first, like self-punishment, it is really more of a self-parenting intervention, where a nurturing part of yourself decides that you are unwilling to be the victim of a tantrum child.

We all know people who seem to remain cheerful and upbeat despite enormous calamities which may have befallen them. Ever wonder how they do it? It's the same answer as in the old story about the first-time visitor to New York who went up to a learned-appearing gentleman and asked, "How do you get to Carnegie Hall?" The answer, of course, was, "Practice, lots of practice!"

What we believe is the most powerful option of all.

Norman Cousins

What's So Funny About an Enema?

Using Humor to Advantage

WARNING: Read at your own risk.
Laughter contained in this chapter.

The purpose of this chapter is to give you a chance to laugh if you'd care to. There are no deep insights contained here — just fun. If you should find some insights, so much the better.

Humor makes many things bearable when we are ill. It distances us from the indignities of diagnosis and treatment. It helps restore our common humanity. It dispels fear. It communicates concern. And it gives us an opportunity to vent anger in a non-confrontive fashion. But best of all, it's fun to laugh and it feels good!

You may or may not find all of the jokes and anecdotes in this chapter funny. People have different tastes in humor. What one person finds funny may not be humorous to another. Cultures and background determine what we find humorous.

But it is not without just cause that we have the expression, "Laughter is the best medicine." The Bible reminds us, "A merry heart makes a cheerful countenance, but low spirits sap a man's strength" (Proverbs 17:22, New English Bible). This long-standing belief is now substantiated with scientific evidence proving that laughter has pain-killing power and predisposes our bodies to a relaxed state in which we can rest and heal better. There are whole conferences now on the Healing Power of Laughter, and some hospitals have developed humor rooms.

Laughter may not be the *best* medicine, but it has to be right up there in the top five. . .even in life-threatening circumstances. How about giving it more room in your life? You can, if determined enough, find something funny in almost anything, even in life-threatening circumstances.

Joe was an older man who was dying of intestinal cancer. He had not had an easy life, a good deal of which had been spent as a heavy drinker. In the last few years with his consistent sobriety came an improved relationship with his oldest daughter.

Their father-daughter relationship had been a stormy one over the years, perhaps accounting for what was now respect and endearment on both sides. In their culture, expression of such feelings as affection were rarely verbal and, then, only indirectly.

Rene arrived one afternoon to find her father exhausted, slipping in and out of alertness. He said, with considerable effort, "Rene, do you know what they did to me?"

"No, Dad. What?"

"Dey gavf me an enema?"

"Oooh, Dad."

"Rene, do you know what an enema iss?"

"Yes, Dad I do."

"O' ya. Any a--hole would!"

They both burst into laughter and began the reminiscing that so often brought him comfort in his last days.

Of course serious illness is serious! Why else would they call it "serious"? That is all the more reason to avail yourself of every advantage — including laughter.

For many people, humor helps disarm fear. If you have cancer, AIDS, or some other life-threatening illness, it is normal to be afraid, feel out of control, at least part of the time. However, if you take an active part in dealing with that fear, you can continue to function under difficult circumstances. Fear is a reasonable response to illness, but should not negate logic.

The story is told of two generals, one older and wiser than the other, the older general functioning as a tutor for the younger one. As they were preparing to go out into mock battle, the older general turned to his aide-de-camp and said, "Fetch me my red tunic!"

A puzzled look came over the younger general's face, and he asked, "Excuse me, General, but why did you ask for your *red* tunic?"

"The reason is quite simple," the older general replied. "In the event I am wounded in battle, I do not want my soldiers to see the blood. That way, they will continue to fight on as soldiers should and not concern themselves with me."

The younger general thought this was a good idea and turned to his aide-de-camp and said, "Fetch me my brown trousers!"

Many of the patients who come to see me have on brown trousers. But their fear doesn't stop them from enjoying a good laugh and even feeling better for it! Humor makes even the worst problem a little more tolerable. The more absurd, the more helpful for some.

Let me tell you about my patient Lynn. She and her husband were able to inject humor into a difficult circumstance, turning a tough day into a memorable one. Lynn was a very refined and lovely lady who had the misfortune to develop widespread breast cancer shortly after marrying. She was thirty-five and enjoyed an active and varied sex life with her husband. Lynn was receiving chemotherapy for her breast cancer and would occasionally develop nausea and vomiting for the twenty-four hours after receiving her medication.

As luck would have it, Lynn and her husband had arranged to host a cocktail party for a visiting dignitary on the same day that she had received her chemotherapy. Her husband returned home to find Lynn attempting to prepare hors d'oeuvres in the kitchen while periodically having to interrupt her labors to rush to the sink to vomit. Not knowing what was happening, he asked her, "What's going on?"

"I forgot that I was scheduled to get my chemo today when we set up this party, and I'm really sick!" she replied while rushing past him to get to the sink.

Being a man of very quick wit, he responded "I guess sex is out of the question then?"

At which point they both burst out laughing.

Lynn continued to vomit discreetly during the cocktail party but each time broke out in laughter remembering her husband's remark, which of course she couldn't share with anyone. It isn't fun to be nauseated by chemotherapy, but it's a lot easier to take if you can laugh at it!

Illness is riddled with difficult and embarrassing experiences, many of which can cause a loss of self esteem.

> Have you heard about the airline stewardess who went to see her doctor and said, "Doctor, I wonder if you can help me? Recently I've been passing a lot of gas. It doesn't smell bad, and it makes no noise, but it embarrasses me nevertheless! There! You see? It happened just now! What do you think we should do about it?"
>
> The doctor stroked his chin thoughtfully, and then said "Well, I think the first thing we had better do is fix your nose!"

Now that we've gotten embarrassing bodily functions out of the way, let's laugh about communication problems. It goes without saying that there are unlimited possibilities for communication difficulties in the realm of illness. Just think about it. Let's start with the doctors! Doctors say what they *don't* mean all the time. When your doctor says, "We did a brain scan and didn't find anything," that is not exactly what was meant. (At least you better hope it wasn't!)

Doctors sometimes fail to realize that patients take things literally, particularly when under stress. I can clearly recall asking a patient, "What brings you to the hospital?" and having him respond, "The bus"!

All human communication is fraught with the possibility of error and misunderstanding and can be misleading, as the following story illustrates:

> Two neighbors, who had a long-standing dispute about their fence line, were seen to be out walking their dogs one day some weeks after their territorial battle had been settled in court. Harold's dog was a giant, vicious German shepherd, while Burt's was a newly acquired, short, squat, nondescript ugly cur. They were both on the same sidewalk approaching each other.

Harold said, "Get off the sidewalk or I'll release my dog!"

Burt replied, "I have as much right to be here as you. Besides, my dog can take on yours any day."

Harold released his dog and Burt did the same. There was an enormous gnashing of teeth, and bits of hair and bone were scattered everywhere. When the dust settled, only Burt's dog was left, sitting quietly with a very broad smile on its mouth.

"What kind of dog is that?" asked Harold.

"To tell the truth. . ." replied Burt, "before it had plastic surgery, it was an alligator."

One of the communication skills most needed in dealing with illness is the ability to see the humor in every situation. Even the overeager helper's efforts are almost funny if you can get the right perspective.

A lady had the misfortune to have one of her relatives pass away suddenly. She attended the viewing at the funeral home and as she stood looking down into the coffin, she said to the funeral director, "Give him some chicken soup!"

The funeral director was astonished and replied, "Madam, this man is dead!"

The lady heard him but still insisted, "Give him some chicken soup!"

The funeral director, thinking the lady was hard of hearing, repeated even louder, "Madam, this man is dead!"

The lady still insisted, "Give him some chicken soup!"

The funeral director was by now becoming a little irritated and shouted, "Lady, this man is stone cold dead!!"

On hearing this, the lady looked at him, shrugged her shoulders, and said, "It couldn't hurt."

(If some of your friends, loved ones, or doctors think some of our ideas in this book are a little crazy — but you don't — just tell them the chicken soup story and say, "It couldn't hurt!")

As we've already discussed in the last chapter, attitude has a great deal to do with outcome.

The story is told about the enthusiastic young American recruit in World War I who arrived in the trenches in France to be informed that there were no more rifles available. "What shall I use for a weapon?" he asked his sergeant.

"Take this stick," said the sergeant, breaking a branch off a nearby bush.

"How do I use it?" asked the recruit.

"Point it at the enemy and say, 'Clickety-click.'"

"Are you sure it will work?" asked the recruit.

"Do you truly believe in our cause?" asked the sergeant.

"Yes I do," responded the recruit.

"Then it'll work" answered the sergeant.

The recruit took his weapon and peered over the edge of the trench to discover that an assault by the enemy had just begun. He pointed his stick at the oncoming soldiers and said, "Clickety-click."

One of the enemy soldiers immediately fell down.

The recruit pointed his stick again and again while dispatching several more enemy soldiers.

Just then he noticed a very large enemy soldier plodding deliberately toward him. He confidently raised his stick and said, "Clickety-click."

But nothing happened.

The enemy soldier continued to march forward. The American recruit tried again. He pointed his stick and said, "Clickety-click."

Again, nothing happened. And now the enemy soldier was even closer.

The recruit tried one more time. He pointed the stick and shouted as loudly as possible, "Clickety-click."

The enemy soldier continued to march slowly forward. As the recruit's helmet was being ground into the dirt by the enemy soldier's boots, he heard the soldier saying to himself, "Tankety-tank, tankety-tank."

Humor can also help us come to terms with painful problems. Grace was a very obese older woman who was referred for severe pain in the stump remaining after her right leg was amputated. She had many grievances directed against the doctors who had previously cared for her, as well as anger resulting from the situation in which she found herself. One day she was sitting in her wheelchair with her amputated stump visible, feeling somewhat self-conscious about being noticed by the other patients, when one of the office staff returned from lunch and noticed her sitting there.

"How are you doing, Grace?" she asked.

"Fine," Grace replied in a soft voice.

"And how are the ballet lessons coming?"

At this point Grace began laughing so hard that she nearly fell out of her wheelchair. All the other patients were laughing too and were waiting for her reply. It didn't take long for Grace to come out with, "Wait 'til you see my tutu!"

This exchange broke the ice, and soon the entire waiting room was involved in conversation with Grace. Now whenever one of the other patients sees Grace, she is usually asked about her tutu, much to her delight.

Perhaps you can find something funny about your own tutu!

How are you going to introduce more humor into your life? Patients have told us that they have started video collections, begun reading children's comic books, or now join their grandchildren in watching Saturday morning cartoons.

How about . . .

- hanging up a sign that reads "TOLL DOOR: NO ADMIT-TANCE WITHOUT A JOKE"?

- doing impersonations of your doctor or a nosy neighbor?

- writing Al in care of LuraMedia and requesting the unedited version of this book?

- developing a list of "one-liners" for surviving embarrassing situations?

- going people watching at a mall?

- sending notes to the kitchen via your food tray?

- hiring a clown?

- becoming a clown?

- going to a kindergarten concert?

What makes humor work? Often it is the timing. You probably have experienced yourself laughing at something at one in the morning that wasn't even funny at four the next afternoon. But mostly it is the relationship between two people that makes something humorous. When we don't understand each other's needs, we have difficulty generating and hearing what is funny. Sure, humor is a defense mechanism sometimes, but we all need some defenses. When both people understand that need, the humor is accepted. It is the understanding, caring context that allows humor to be so pointed, so unique to a relationship. Humor is not a universal language, but it is spoken more commonly than you might suspect. How about trying it more often?

Life does not cease to be funny when people die, any more than it ceases to be serious when people laugh.

George Bernard Shaw

The Flowers Were Lovely,
But We Really Needed a Casserole

Using Your Support System Effectively

One day an elderly couple driving along a main avenue met an ambulance racing in the opposite direction with its siren going full volume. As it passed the husband said, "Honey, they're playing our song!" They were both relieved that this time it was not coming for them.

Chronic and/or life-threatening illness is a varied song. For some it is the blues, for others a banal hymn, for others a never ending ballad of adventure, and for yet others, the "Battle Hymn of the Republic." Whatever it is for you, it is never a solo. That is not to say that you may not feel drowned out by the chorus, or on center stage without your lines. Whatever the circumstances, illness is experienced by one person but it influences the lives of many.

All kinds of people can be part of your support system. Many people tell us that their illness is a time when they find out who really cares.

What kind of care do you want? Do you expect? Do you need? We all have our own lists of "If you really cared, you would..."

- "If you really cared, you would come to see me in the hospital."

- "If you really cared, you would find time to take me places."

- "If you really cared, you wouldn't pity me."

- "If you really cared, you wouldn't expect so much of me."

- "If you really cared, you would be upfront with me."
- "If you really cared, you would respect my privacy."

. . .and on it goes.

There seem to be three kinds of patients. The *opportunists* are those who think that being ill is a license to demand all the things they never had the guts to ask for before. The *tyrants* are those who feel that, because they were in a position to order people around in the "well world," they should have the same privilege in the "ill world." Both of these types seem to assume that once they have an illness, everyone else has forfeited all rights to being treated humanly and all rights to having their needs met. No one really knows if these people are covering their fear through their attempts at controlling everything and everyone, or if they are, at some level, relieved to have a legitimate reason to be taken care of without having to admit the need.

The other extreme is the *apologizers* who are chronically apologizing for their condition, demonstrating they feel they have *no* rights because they are ill. Their apologies get boring after a while. The more frustrating aspect of relating to them, however, is that they will not make their needs clear, and their support system is left feeling obliged but not knowing what they "should do" or whether they have done enough.

If you are the type of person who apologizes each time you make a request, we suggest you spend some extra time in the chapter "Pardon Me and I'll Pardon You: Dealing with Guilt" (page 148). At some point you have to look in the mirror and decide whether you are going to go through life apologizing for having an illness. Because you have different needs does not mean you have to apologize for getting them met. It gets a bit tacky if you are always saying, "Oh, I'm sorry, but would you mind if. . ."

For most of us, our list of sensitivities goes on. Most of us don't like being vulnerable or needy in front of others. That's not surprising. Very few people find it easy to tolerate being unable to move themselves, unable to make their car payments, unable to make love, or unable to do the basics in life. No one is expecting you to like it, but neither do people want to be a target for your feelings about everything. They just want to help. How many times has someone finished a conversation with, "If there is anything we can do, just call"? And how many times have you called?

When you have finally decided to accept the offer for help, it can be pretty disconcerting when the same people who sounded so available suddenly have a list of reasons why they can't help. What do you do then? Tell yourself they don't care or that you aren't worthy? Feel worse than before you asked? It usually takes a person aback for a short time, but you do have the option of moving beyond your disappointment or anger. *Their inability to help tells you something about THEIR world. It is not a statement about YOUR worth.* If you want revenge, get well! If you don't want them to feel badly, get your need met elsewhere so they don't have to feel guilty. Tell them you hope their world is less cluttered soon and phone the next person. If you want to create a little puzzlement, ask them sincerely if there is anything you can help them with.

You will probably encounter a variety of types of caregiving. The two most common mistakes helpers make is that they help too much or they help too little. They have to be trained. Some, in an attempt to respect your privacy and independence, leave you in an emotional vacuum, which, in turn, encourages you to attempt tasks you logically might better have someone else perform. This type overstays a visit by twice your energy, brings you work from the office a day after surgery, and watches you take ten minutes to reach something they could pass to you in a moment. They just don't want you to feel they are pampering you. They are usually highly successful. Try to remember they may be the kind of person who would themselves not want, or are afraid, to be pampered a little. That's nicer than thinking they are just insensitive clods.

Ironically, compassionate care is not as available from those we count on as we might think or expect. Patients have all kinds of experiences that make them shake their heads in disbelief when it comes to caring. I think of the woman who was out for lunch. An old friend, who knew she had a poor prognosis and was on chemo, came over smiling and asked how she was. When the woman stated quite objectively that she was having trouble with nausea following her chemo, the friend quickly replied, "Oh, do you have to talk about something like that at lunch?"

On the other hand, some people will smother you. You know the type: the person who treats you as if it's your brain that is not working, rather than your heart or lungs. If they take you for lunch, they want to order for you. They won't tell you any of the gossip at work, and they use a tone of voice that would lull a four-year-old.

Common sense dictates that you ask for help from persons who are likely to be able to assist. Everyone has his or her own strengths. Tammy recognized this in an incident during her illness. Her closest friend called the hospital to say that she would not be coming to see her until Tammy was much better. She said she just did not do well visiting people who were ill. Tammy was a little miffed and disappointed. However, this same person sent flowers and later arranged a welcome home surprise party. She really could not handle hospitals. She knew her own limits.

When people do not know their own limits, the experience can be devastating. Jane realized this when her friend visited and was so taken aback by her change in appearance that he threw up in the kidney basin. A fine hello that was!

People are often only as awkward at helping as you are at asking. Most people will help if they can, particularly if you are able to be very specific about what you want or do not want. Men, in particular, tend to be more comfortable if they know specifically what is being asked. That's not so surprising: Women often get more experience in caregiving than men.

But before you can be clear about your requests, you have to wrestle with several questions:

- "What can I realistically do for myself?"

- "With what would I *like* help?"

- "With what do I *need* help?"

We said this was a book of recipes. Here is one for "Getting What You Need":

1. Be honest. Refuse to plead or apologize.

2. Say, "I need..."

3. Complete the sentence by saying what it is that you need. When appropriate, allow the person the option of being unable to meet the request.

4. Provide any necessary or helpful instructions.

5. Thank the person.

Here are some examples of what we mean:

- "I need my bedside tray. I would appreciate it if you would move it over here, please. It has a catch on the side to release it for moving. . . . Thanks."

- "I need my left side supported when I walk. Are you willing to do that? Here is how. . ."

- "I need these letters mailed. Would you be willing to mail them for me?"

Notice that we are not suggesting you spend a lot of time explaining *why* you have a particular need. In some cases it is logical to provide such information, but we don't suggest long, ingratiating explanations.

Joyce, a beautiful single parent of a fourteen-year-old, had an advanced disease that made even the daily tasks extremely difficult. She wanted to be at home as long as possible, but social services could provide only four hours of help each week, and she had no extended family near her home. Joyce had a number of friends, but very few of them knew each other. They all worried that they were not doing enough and yet were all feeling burdened with the extra weight they were carrying.

With Joyce's permission, her daughter and eight friends met one evening. With the help of a counselor, every need and problem was identified — right down to the fact that Joyce never seemed to have quarters for the washing machine. Meals, grocery shopping, banking, transportation to treatments, the need for humor, some "normal living and playing with others" for her daughter were all part of the needs list. One need which Joyce wanted to handle for herself was disseminating information and handling her phone calls. She agreed and lived up to the necessity of limiting the amount of time of her calls. She learned to say, "I need to go now so I don't use all of my energy." One need initially went unexpressed. When asked whether she had any spiritual needs, somewhat to everyone's surprise the answer was, "Yes." One of the group accepted the task to arrange for a pastoral counselor. When each person left the meeting with a task, no one felt over-burdened, Joyce's needs were covered, and each person felt they were contributing something of importance.

There are families by nature and families by choice. Families by choice often work just as well. Joyce's chosen family worked together to meet Joyce's needs until her death. It takes guts to do what Joyce did, to say, "Here are my needs. Can you help? What I can offer back is my courage, my will to live, and my ability to listen." What Joyce gave in return more than offset the few hours that each person contributed. They felt privileged to be able to help.

But what if you don't have family or friends around you? Because your brother is in Florida, your sister in Saskatchewan, and you have just moved into town doesn't mean that there is no one to care. It does mean it will take a few phone calls to find out who and what is available. It also means you have to accept that this is a time when you are going to meet new people on a basis that you would not have preferred. There are agencies that can help. There is a lot of love in any community. The biggest hurdle is getting over asking for help. If the help was for someone else, would you have as much trouble asking?

Take a look at your own situation. Close your eyes and get out your imaginary notebook and picture the word "NEEDS" at the top of the page. Notice what appears under this heading. On another page, imagine the heading "SUPPORT SYSTEM." Notice what names appear on that list. Do any of them surprise you? Beside each person's name, notice that there is an indication of what kinds of needs they can help you meet. There is everything from laughter to casseroles. (You may want to transfer what you see to an actual notebook.)

Notice what you *cannot* count on from some people. No point in counting on a heart-to-heart talk about life and death from Elroy. He is scared of his own shadow emotionally. He would do a thousand errands for you, though. Notice there is someone who can even take care of the pets. There is likely a combination of medical people, family, and friends available to help you.

Go back to your list of needs. Are there any needs that are still unmet when you have gone over what people in your world can do? How can you get those needs met? Who can you even *express* those needs to?

Close your imaginary notebook and turn on an imaginary television. See someone (it could be you) with the same unmet need in the same situation that you are in. Watch the program. See how the need gets met. Is the person you are watching changing the nature of the need, making it different in some way? Perhaps the person is having a meeting with someone about it.

Someone in your world will know a person or a way that your need can be met.

Using this imaginary television technique, one mother saw herself as the executive of her family, calling a meeting, handing out file folders and an agenda, and discussing not only her needs but also the needs of the whole family during this time of stress. She went on to actually hold that meeting and was the self-declared chief executive of her family throughout her illness. The shareholders were initially puzzled but came to like the new form of management. It included divisions of labor, meals according to menus, schedules of who would be where and when. Everyone gained. The company flourished.

Your image may be very different. Let it unfold. There is a creative side of you that will come up with solutions if you will focus on the problem — without judgment, without fear, without anger.

 You can do it with a little help from your friends.

In Case of Fire, Use the Stairs

Developing New Skills and Maximizing Old Ones

Perhaps you have noticed this sign next to elevators in many high-rise buildings: "In case of fire, use the stairs!" Elevator call buttons are heat-activated, and in the event of fire, the elevator would stop at every floor. Therefore, it's necessary to find alternative means of getting out of the building.

So, too, it is necessary in the case of serious illness to know what the alternatives are and to develop new resources. It is time to take a skills inventory. What skills do you already have? What skills do you need to develop? Human beings are amazingly versatile creatures and develop creative solutions to the most perplexing problems.

At a diving meet a young lady on the visiting team caught my attention. She was diving very well and had received some excellent scores. The interesting thing was that she had no arms! Apparently she had been born without them. This did not seem to limit her in any fashion whatever. She was able to use the diving board as effectively as any other diver and even was able to attain sufficient height to perform complex dives. (And I *know* how essential arms are to attaining the correct momentum and height for the dives!)

Watching her get out of the pool with confidence and ingenuity was rather like watching the evolution of a human being from a water-dwelling to a land-dwelling creature. Needless to say, I was very impressed and proud of the whole human species.

As I was watching the young lady perform, I overheard one of the other divers talking to her parents. "Pretty remarkable, isn't she?" said the parents. "But what's really remarkable is to watch her putting on her bathing suit!" replied the diver.

Imagine how much more difficult any perplexing problem you

have would be if you didn't have any arms. Perhaps you have arms but are lacking some other coping skill. The good news is that you can acquire new skills which will solve your problem.

Looking at things from a different perspective often enables us to see solutions that were there all the time, but which we were unable to see before! We all tend to overlook the obvious. How many times have you gone around the house looking for your glasses which you had pushed up onto the top of your head? How many times have you searched the house for your keys, only to discover that they were in the door? Never? Well, I have!

Sometimes it pays to step back from a problem in order to get a better perspective on resolving it.

Have you ever had your car stuck in the snow? No? How about mud or sand? I thought so! One of the first things you learn under those circumstances is to put the car into reverse to get enough momentum to go forward and get out of the rut you were in.

How can you get enough momentum to get out of the rut you might find yourself in with your illness? How about doing *one* thing differently?

June is a lovely lady who had a severe fear of flying. She wanted to accompany her husband on a well-deserved holiday to Hawaii. June had been in an airplane before, but it was a white-knuckle experience that neither she nor her husband wished to repeat. Her fear of flying was rooted in a fear of dying. You see, June felt that if she died, she would never go to heaven because she was unworthy. Her unworthiness was rooted in her childhood experiences that had to do with never being perfect in her mother's eyes. Naturally, as a human being, she had imperfections like all the rest of us, but she felt she couldn't forgive herself the tiniest imperfection.

As you might expect, June was an excellent housekeeper. Nothing in her home could ever be the slightest bit out of order. She even used a tape measure to make sure that the ashtray on her living room coffee table was exactly in the center of the table at all times.

We began to help her change by extracting a promise that she would allow the ashtray on her coffee table to be off center during her next party which was coming up soon. If anyone even *seemed* to notice that it was off center, she had permission to restore it to the exact center of the table immediately!

Naturally, no one noticed. We knew we were really making

progress when June came to the office with a big smile on her face. When asked why she was smiling, she said, "I was just locking the front door to come here when I heard the phone ringing. And I didn't go back inside to answer it!"

Not long after that, she was able to tell her mother that she loved her, and miraculously her mother responded, "I love you too!"

June's fear of flying vanished shortly thereafter, and we got a nice postcard from Hawaii!

Some changes we choose. Some changes are imposed on us. You may not have done anything to have a change imposed on you; nevertheless, change may be required. What small change could you make that might be the beginning of a whole new approach to your problems?

How about telling someone that you love them? No, no, not the mail carrier! Someone you've known for a long time and who has been a true friend. I've never known of anyone whose feelings were hurt by being told that they were loved.

(Ah, why not! If you think it would be a good idea, tell the mail carrier, too!)

Change may be a key to your well-being. New skills may be required. But what about the *old* skills, the things that you already know you do well? It's time to get them out, dust them off, and put them to use under these new circumstances. They can be invaluable.

Who you are can help. The positive parts of your personality are assets: your sense of humor, your caring for others, even your stubbornness, if you use it well. Your ability to make decisions and set priorities, your ability to solve problems, your ability to help others with their feelings are all personal and interpersonal skills that help in an illness.

Other very practical skills are not to be ignored. Being able to knit while you wait for appointments is one skill you probably have not considered. Mary, who came for regular treatments, managed to complete seventeen sweaters before the end of her program. She felt good about having done the sweaters and was not resentful toward the medical staff for the waiting periods.

Letter-writing, food preparation, reading, golfing, computer skills — the list is endless. Think of every activity that you feel capable of doing. Each of them involves a skill. Those skills might be applicable in the management of your illness. Perhaps you have never thought of telling stories to your grandchildren or your ability to organize a car wash as skills. They are!

Once you have developed new skills and polished up your old ones, there remains one more skill to develop: that of trying new approaches and being able to tolerate making mistakes. If you are not making enough mistakes, you are not trying out enough new ideas. We may not have written the perfect book, but it sure beats sitting around saying, "You know, we really should write a book some day!" The best part of being willing to make mistakes is succeeding at something that you did not know you could do and being able to take well-deserved pride in yourself!

A ship in port is safe, but that's not what ships are built for.

Grace Hopper

Riches on the Inside

Strengths Money Can't Buy

What about money?

What about it? It's only money! Easy to say, not so easy to feel. Financial pressures can be very real, particularly if there is little or no insurance. Money *does* help. It can buy services, and services ease part of the burden. But, in and of itself, money does not make you rich. We have observed wealthy people die in emotional poverty, and financially impoverished persons experience great richness. The important thing is to get whatever financial help you need and refuse to be embarrassed. You may be richer than you think!

Emily was a woman in her early sixties who lived with her daughter and grandson, Mark. Emily helped with childcare and was adored by Mark. They had very little in terms of material things. Emily's disease was obviously advancing, but she often found time and energy to roam the halls of the hospital, comforting those whom she thought of as less fortunate. Her roommate plagued Emily with the distress of deciding how much of her large estate to leave to each of her sons, neither of whom had come to visit her. When I asked Emily how she was doing with her roommate, Emily smiled in her gentle way and replied, "Well, I guess some people are rich on the outside and some people are rich on the inside. I guess if it's gotta be one or the other, I feel lots richer."

Emily had inner resources. There was something about her spirit that was strong and gentle and uniquely Emily. In our work we are often sustained by the magnitude of the courage and hope expressed by our patients. In even the most disconcerting circumstances, the one remarkable source of hope and inspiration is the profoundness of the human spirit.

This book could not be complete without raising the topic of the spiritual, yet no topic gave us greater qualms about writing (and there are definite difficulties with being witty about this most intimate dimension of our lives). Answers to questions in the realm of the spiritual are always personal. Einstein said, "It is only to the individual that a soul is given." Each person, at some level, wrestles with what life and death are about. Some accept the limits of human knowledge and ask no further. Others take the leap of faith. Most, at some point, search for meaning. We make no assumption that one spiritual journey or pathway is more enlightening than another. We would hope for validity in the statement of Kahlil Gibran who said, "God made Truth with many doors to welcome every believer who knocks on them."

Some activities and relationships clearly strengthen the human spirit; others clearly diminish it. What nourishes the soul or spirit of one person may not help another. Each of us has a unique way of expressing our spirit. For some, it may be the memory of an experience in which they felt connected with the universe. Graeme, my colleague, described it this way:

> "I used to think that a good life is a long life. If you could get your three score and ten, that's a privilege. I want that for myself, but I no longer have that necessarily as the ideal. The essential thing is the quality of time that I live. I don't know how you measure that. I think it could possibly be measured in moments. If you have a few moments in your life that are real highlights and deeply meaningful, you could die feeling satisfied and peaceful.
>
> "I will always remember being at 13,000 feet behind Mt. Annapurna in a little temple in Nepal which is both a Hindu and Buddhist pilgrimage point, listening to my Walkman play "Chariots of Fire" and just standing there watching the mountains. That was spectacular. That was one of those moments. I was almost overwhelmed with the beauty.
>
> "There has been a change in my spirit. I love more deeply. I appreciate more deeply. I bask in the sun more fully. I take time to smell the roses, to really see the sunsets. Likewise, with my relationships. Looking from

the top of Annapurna, the boundaries between me and
everything else were a lot less clear. I felt connected
with everything. I can't say I live from that spot very
often, but I'm more aware of it. The biggest change in
my spirit is that I am less afraid."

Jean, a woman in her mid-fifties, moved out to her cabin for the
last year of her life. It was there that she felt that her spirit could be
free. She felt a deep connection with the earth and was determined
to see all four seasons from the window overlooking the lake. She
recorded her experiences in a journal throughout the year. I share with
you one excerpt:

"It's lovely here — incredible blue sky and cumulus
clouds across a steel grey lake — marvelous thunder and
lightning and the lawn is covered in hail and snow. Fire
is going and the music is excellent. Marvelous storm.
The world here tonight has every possible mood."

Others have described the sense of spiritual in terms of their relationships. Alice speaks of "real connections":

"A real connection happens almost without words. There
are words, but the real connection happens at the heart
level. When I have a real connection, I feel satisfied. I
feel nurtured. I feel enriched. I have to be open for it
without grabbing for it. I feel like an open vessel. You
can't have a deep connection without sharing. . . . We
can call on something greater than ourselves, whatever
that might be. You can call it spirit, energy, consciousness, love. I call it God."

Stan spoke of his spirit in this way:

"I don't always have the power and strength to do what I
want. It fades on me, and I get terribly tired. I get
somewhat depressed. On those days I don't have a lot of
willpower, but for the most part, I have will from inner
depths. I don't really know where it comes from. I've just
got it because I am a strong person and a very tough person.

I also have fantastic family support from friends and acquaintances, too. That's the source of most of my strength.

"The only thing I know is to keep fighting and keep struggling. I've seen people who didn't. Maybe there was no struggle left for them. I'm not sure. I will never know. I just know that in the time I have, I want to be able to live something resembling a normal life. I want to spend time with my family without them feeling that I'm an invalid, that I'm a drag on the family. I want to see my boys grow up. I feel I have a lot of things I want to do. I'm not ready to die, and I'm not ready to become a total invalid."

Some report the power of prayer in their lives, while others attribute a quieting of spirit to meditation. Del reported the apparent profoundness of "soul searching." It seemed to be a turning point in his illness:

"Things turned pretty ugly at one point. My lungs got worse. I ended up on oxygen. I was in and out of the hospital. Then, more in than out . . . I had to be taken off chemo. I developed shingles. What else could go wrong! I recall thinking, 'Why am I bothering to continue to live?' I thought, 'This is so difficult, I can't believe it!' I had never felt worse physically. I couldn't eat anything. I didn't have a vein left that would take an intravenous.

"There was a point where I had to do some soul searching. 'Am I going to get better or am I just going to die here?' That night I seemed to go downhill. The medical situation worsened. My veins were nonexistent. My blood was dropping off. I was having trouble staying oriented. They had to put in a catheter. I couldn't even reach my cassette player to play my tapes. [He is an avid user of meditation and relaxation tapes.]

"The next morning something was right. The head of the clinic came in and said, 'I think you have turned a corner.' Ten days later I was out of the hospital."

For others, spirituality has always been more along the lines of a traditional faith. Pat says simply:

"I have always had my church. That has meant a great deal to me. My faith still does. I feel that it has carried me through. I've always felt that God was there. I find myself talking to God constantly. As far back as I can remember, I've been asking, 'Now, God, why this?' or 'Well, you know, God, this is coming up and we need a little bit of help.' "

There is a paradox about speaking of inner resources: Part of the strengthening of one's inner resources is a sense of being connected to and strengthened by something or someone outside of one's self.

How do you strengthen your spirit? We recognize several themes among people, regardless of the specific, or nonspecific, theology which they hold.

Every person has something that has the potential to strengthen the spirit. We have noticed that people with the kind of spirit that is life-giving have an interest outside of themselves, particularly outside of their illness and hassles.

What strengthens you? Is it nature — a beautiful sunset? watching a seedling sprout? enjoying the season? Certain people — a grandchild? a particular visitor? an inspiring author? Certain regular practices — meditation? prayer? attendance at worship service? long distance running? Certain objectives — a particular task to be completed? a dream yet to unfold? a lesson yet to be learned? a purpose unfulfilled? Notice and cultivate whatever nourishes you. There doesn't have to be a reason *why*. Our spirit is not a rational, problem-solving part of us. *It simply is*. It does not judge. It will move toward health if you will notice what soothes and strengthens it.

A nonjudgmental or loving attitude, not to be confused with passive, appears to strengthen more than a condemning or critical attitude does.

The value of sharing also seems apparent in the strengthening of the spirit. Some people can share and speak of their inner world freely. For others, it is a totally private world. Regardless of style, it is an important world — a world that helps and heals.

A nurse reported this memory of a patient who will always be endeared to her. Sam was a tough motorcycle gang member. He spoke very little of what was going on inside him. One day he asked the nurse if she would like to see his "leathers." She quietly affirmed that she would, a little cautiously, as she did not know what "leathers" were. He lifted from the clothing locker the leather leggings he had worn while riding his motorcycle and laid them on the bed. He said simply, "My friend gave me those. I want to be buried in them." He was sharing a little of his inner world, a little about who had been important to him, a little of what had strengthened his spirit.

Kahlil Gibran said, "To be closer to God, be closer to people." Is there someone who could be your spiritual partner — someone with whom you could discuss life and death and meaning? It needs to be someone you can trust. It will likely be someone who you feel strongly will share some of his or her spiritual journey with you. This is often not a spouse or a close family member. You needn't feel you are betraying the family if you choose someone outside of the family for this role. If you do not have someone like this, you will need to decide whether you will reach out in this way. Are you ready to trust?

Trust is the other observation we have in terms of spirituality. People who have strong spirits appear to trust something. Their ability to let go and trust their inner resources paradoxically gives them more control over their lives. It is amazing in our world of frenzied living that we trust elevators, traffic lights, strangers operating on our bodies, air travel, and medications, but we have difficulty trusting the oldest human resource — the human spirit.

We have also observed a number of themes in terms of what diminishes the human spirit. It does not seem related to the specific kind of beliefs one holds. We have seen many an agnostic die peacefully, satisfied with their lives, surrounded by loving families. We have also seen people with religious beliefs die in fear, disappointed in their lives, and alone with a bedside table stacked high with devotionals and testimonials which suggest they are studying for their finals.

A common pitfall is one which includes believing that illness is a punishment. Often this gets extended to include the idea that illness is just the beginning of a sentence which will be continued in hell. Carried to extreme, this can lead to a person feeling so unworthy they feel they do not deserve to be healed, or that if any healing is to occur, it must come directly from God.

Eileen was a well-educated woman who insisted that cancer was her punishment for being an inadequate wife and mother. Since she had chosen to work outside the home, Eileen decided that God was punishing her and that, since God gave her the disease, God could also cure her. But she was convinced that this would not happen because she was not worthy. She refused treatment. To observers, it looked very much like death was preferable to taking charge of her life. In Eileen's view she had, at forty-six, failed to be a perfect person and therefore deserved to die.

She did.

The opposite can happen as well. Bernie Siegel in *Love, Medicine and Miracles* adapts an old story to make the point:

> "A man with cancer is told by his primary physician he'll be dead in an hour. He runs to the window, looks up at the sky, and says, 'God, save me.' Out of the blue comes that wonderful melodious voice, saying, 'Don't worry, my son. I will save you.' The man climbs back into bed, feeling reassured.
>
> "[A surgeon calls and says,] 'If I operate in an hour, I can save you.' 'No, thanks,' [replies] the man, 'God will save me.' Then an oncologist, a radiation therapist, and a nutritional therapist all tell him, 'We can save you.' 'I don't need you. God will save me,' was his reply to all of them.
>
> "In an hour the man dies. When he gets to heaven, he walks up to God and says, 'What happened? You said you'd save me, and here I am, dead.'
>
> " 'You dumbbell. I sent you a surgeon, an oncologist, a radiation therapist, and a nutritional therapist.' "

Still others feel betrayed or abandoned. Perhaps, more realistically, confused and resentful. They feel they struck a bargain and God didn't hold up the other half of the bargain. They feel they have lived a good and devout life, and now God has denied them their just reward of a comfortable retirement or a normal life span. Unfortunately, a belief in God does not guarantee immunity to disease or struggle.

Nor does a belief in God ensure that one will have all the answers and none of the feelings. Many people find it difficult when they realize they are feeling angry at God. When they experience abandonment, they become afraid their faith won't see them through. They become afraid of the very feelings God put in the original design.

Our emotional systems are no less miraculous than our physical systems or the universe itself. Every feeling is there for a purpose, to help us deal with something. We can assume that, like the poster says, "God don't make junk," and, therefore, all emotions are created with a function. When a person decides to believe in God (or whatever name you would use), God doesn't reach down and disconnect the feelings that make us uncomfortable.

Some people are afraid to be angry with God. Now, we are not talking about a fragile relationship! A little anger from you isn't going to upset anyone except you. Who are you kidding? You can't hide feelings from God! The other nice thing is that God keeps things confidential. You can tell God anything and not another soul will know.

Check your expectations of your beliefs about a power greater than you. Do any of these sound familiar?

- "If I believe, I should never be afraid."

- "If I believe, I should never feel alone."

- "If I believe, I should be a model of adjustment."

- "If I believe, I should never feel far away from God."

- "If I believe, I should never waver in my faith."

Should! Should! Should!

A teenager once put it nicely. He said, "I have been should on all my life." If you feel "should on," it's not God. God accepts our limits.

Unfortunately, not all *people* are as understanding. We have seen lots of examples of how UNhelpful well-meaning, religious people can be. Unfortunately, being a believer creates no immunity to being insensitive to the needs of others.

There was the mother who refused to forgive her son for living with a woman she didn't like. He was on his way to surgery for reoccurrence of cancer. Going to surgery with your mother angry with you is not great.

In another instance I found it difficult to watch a young man of eighteen years die a painful death with his parents admonishing him until the last moments for not praying hard enough.

Ministers also are not exempt from committing insensitivities. A good minister is like a good doctor. Get one you can talk with and who you feel has a sense of your needs. The minister called to the deathbed of one of my patients will likely *not* qualify!

Alex had had a very difficult illness and one of the rare painful deaths I have ever seen. His family had suffered as observers to the process. Alex finally died one morning at six a.m. attended by his exhausted family. The pastor was called and arrived at seven-thirty. He said prayers and told the children that their father had not died, that he had just gone away. He excused himself at eight o'clock, as he was attending university classes of some sort. His parting words to us all were, "Have a good day." It took Alex's wife a very long time to let the memory of that insensitivity fade. It only takes a few insensitive words at the wrong moment to diminish the human spirit.

A belief in God holds a complete form of hope, but for many people, a difficult one to test. Faith is a gift. Not everyone has it, nor does everyone reach out in that direction, even under dire circumstances.

A young man was hiking in the beautiful Canadian Rockies and was admiring the magnificent view. As he walked near a precipice, he failed to notice that he was walking on an overhang. When it gave way, he was fortunate enough to catch himself on a protruding old tree root. He hung precariously and with great difficulty, well aware that when his strength gave out he would plummet to an unwelcome end thousands of feet below. Needless to say, action was called for.

After a quick perusal of the situation, it was clear to him that efforts to save himself, beyond simply holding on, were out of the question. He yelled with full force of the panic he felt, "Is anyone out there?"

A voice that seemed to come from everywhere and from nowhere rumbled, "I am here, my son. I am God. Let go and you will be saved."

The doubtful hiker, after a moment of reflection, yelled with only slightly less despair, "Is anyone else out there?"

If you are in that group of people who say, "I am not sure," think about consulting a member of the clergy or someone you trust. The conversations of any clergyperson and yourself are confidential. If this is a very private aspect of your life, you might take the advice of a woman who put it this way: "I *pray* as if everything is up to God. I *behave* as if everything is up to me."

Don't believe that prayers are answered? Joe was skeptical, too. Matter of fact he wasn't much interested in anything except his enema. The pastoral care visitor was visiting seventy-eight- year-old Joe shortly after Joe had had a stroke. His mental abilities had been impaired by the trauma. Speech was difficult and he wasn't very "with it." But he was "with it" enough that when the pastoral care visitor asked if he would like a little prayer, Joe replied, "Just wanna enema. I'm prayin' for the doctor to come." No more were the words out of his mouth than the doctor appeared at the end of the hall. Astonished, Joe's eyes showed his delight with the seeming power of prayer.

We have seen many people with that "Peace that passeth all under-standing." It is worth looking into. Can several million people be wrong? There would be no harm in reading a bit, or having a confidential chat with a friend or clergyperson of your choice.

Part of the difficulty is that you might not recognize God. The following story was found in a church:

> One night a man had a dream. He dreamt he was walking along the beach with the Lord. Across the sky flashed scenes from his life. For each scene he noticed two sets of footprints in the sand. One belonged to him, and one belonged to the Lord.
>
> When the last scene had flashed before him, he looked back at the footprints and saw that many times along the path there was only one set of footprints in the sand. He also noticed that this happened during the lowest and the saddest times in his life. This really bothered him, and he questioned the Lord.
>
> "Lord, you said that once I decided to follow you, you would never leave me, and that you would walk all the way with me. But I noticed that during the troublesome times of my life, there was only one set of

footprints. I don't understand. Why, when I needed you the most, did you desert me?"

The Lord replied, "My precious child, I love you and would never leave you. During your times of suffering, where you see only one set of footprints, it was then that I carried you."

 As eternity is reckoned, there's a lifetime in a second.

Piet Heim

SECTION 4

COMMUNICATION SKILLS

Keeping the Channels Open

Please Hear What I'm Not Saying

Communication Pitfalls

Phyllis was forty-nine. She had raised three children practically on her own. She had been looking forward to having time and things for herself. Instead, she was in the advanced stages of a chronic illness. She had been thought of as a very adequate lady, but about three weeks after her admission to hospital, she was reported as getting very edgy and cranky with staff. She was reluctant to discuss with me what was bothering her. I respected her privacy and added that I would drop off some crayons and paper, just in case, in the privacy of a moment, she might feel like attempting to portray something of what she was feeling. She would be free to share it or keep it to herself. She looked at me as if I was talking a foreign language but said that it would be fine to leave the materials.

A day later she was eager to show me her picture. It was black on white, showing a simple, round-shaped face with eyes that conveyed abandonment. The mouth was virtually expressionless. Below were written the words, "Ronna, please hear what I'm not saying."

In the time that followed she told of her struggle over the years, and now her struggle with the illness. She was tired of hearing how well she had coped. She wanted some recognition that she felt cheated. She wanted permission *not* to be adequate for at least a few days in the last days of her life.

Phyllis initially had been caught in a common communication pitfall. She wanted people to know what she needed without expressing her needs. The more you rely on the mindreading ability of those who care for you, the more likely you will fall into a communication pitfall. This is a time when clarity of communication in your relationships is especially important.

We have a relationship with everyone in our world — our parents, friends, dentist, doctor, and grandkids. If we are fortunate, we also have a special person in our lives, someone with whom we live and of whom we expect more than we do of the others because we have an agreement, spoken or unspoken, to care. For many, that person is a spouse; for others, it is a chosen partner. For some, the relationship is stable; for others, it is less established and more vulnerable. But even a stable relationship needs a little reassurance once in a while.

> At every twenty-fifth anniversary the story is told of
> the wife who wanted to hear the words "I love you"
> from her husband on their anniversary. He was an
> amiable but gruff fellow who wasn't much for talking
> about feelings. After some cajoling, he succumbed to her
> pressure by saying, "I told ya twenty-five years ago I
> loved you. If anything changes, I'll let ya know."

Well, illness *does* change a relationship! This chapter will give you a kaleidoscope view of the most common communication/relationship problems surrounding illness that we have observed. If you know about them, you can prevent them; and if you can spot them, then you can decide if you want to change anything.

You need to know that this is NOT the chapter on how to rectify the difficulties; we're talking here only about being able to *spot* the problems. If you finish the chapter with sweaty palms, you might want to turn immediately to the next chapter, "Getting the Message Across" (page 97), for some remedies. (This book is not a novel. You can read it in whatever order you want.)

Relationship problems can begin well before the diagnosis of an illness. There obviously can be long-standing difficulties in families or groups of people long before illness arrives. Not every family is the "Family of the Year." There are cranky old uncles, delinquent adolescents, gossipy neighbors, overindulgent parents, and demanding landlords on every street. They do not change a lot just because someone gets ill. The only difference you will probably notice is that they will get crankier, more delinquent, nosier, more indulgent, and more demanding.

We would like to say that there are wonderful transformations in people when they or someone they love gets ill . . . but we did agree to say things as we saw them. We don't want to be totally pessimistic; we just don't want you to hope for the unlikely — although it is possible.

WARNING: Sometimes when you're ill, the best transformation you can hope for among the people around you is that the difficult people will stop visiting.

You may not want to hear that statement. But at least if you know this might be true, you have the option of letting go of unrealistic expectations of people and avoiding disappointment. If someone is surprisingly sensitive, think what a pleasure it will be to write us and say, "You folks were wrong. Stanley came through."

One couple had to face a terminal diagnosis only months after they had decided that they would not get a divorce. They had decided to stay together more for convenience than because of good feelings. Then illness was added to their situation. When the woman's husband announced that he had cancer and was dying, her reaction was, "What are you trying to do to me?" They agreed to make the best out of a difficult situation and to be at least friends throughout the experience. They did it! Too bad they had wasted the years of friendship that could have been.

Another couple described their relationship as a piece of driftwood. Until it was under pressure, they had not even noticed that it had cracks in it.

Take a moment here to check. If you are healthy, in a partnership, and reading this book, you may wish to ask yourself this question: "Are there any signs in my relationship that, if I got ill, I would have to wonder about whether or not I was loved?"

During an illness, there are so many things that need to be done; the extra burden can strain any relationship. If you attempt to remain independent and not burden others, you may find yourself overextending your energy. If you are like most of us, you will then become cranky, exhausted, and/or discouraged. This starts an unfortunate cycle. You withdraw from people who, in turn, feel they have to help which, in turn, makes you more determined than ever to stay independent, which makes you more tired. This routine can get pretty destructive.

Sometimes the opposite happens. Some people take the attitude that, "Now that I am sick, I am a child. YOU do everything. . .as long as it is what I want and the way I want it!"

But the truth is, it's not what you do or do not do that matters.

It's how you handle the *differences in expectations* between how you and the people caring for you think things should be done.

Everything takes energy. To redistribute the energy in your life and still arrange for what has to be done requires the ability to communicate. We all communicate better if we feel safe, if we feel competent, and if we know what we are trying to ask or say. During an illness there are decisions to be negotiated about roles, information, and feelings. It's time to be negotiating how you and the people in your world are going to handle things.

When your illness prevents you from doing certain things, there is the problem of who is going to do them. And how will they *feel* about doing them? Do they also get told that the rules have changed, or should they just *know* what to do because they love you? Perhaps they can enroll in a mind-reading course and major in telepathy. Do they get to take part in any of the decision-making about how things will change? After all, their lives are being changed by the circumstances, too.

Which things do you want to keep trying to do? What can you do that others might have been doing before? How are you and they going to handle the feelings involved in all of these changes?

Oh, yes, the feelings. You were probably hoping that you could be one of the few who handles this illness stuff without blinking an eye. But since you are not brain dead, you will have to deal with those annoying reminders that you are human. Avoiding feelings, or dealing with them insensitively, will just create more troubles. The people who care for you, including your medical team, are human, too. They feel, too. Sadness, anger, and discouragement are not restricted to the patient's experience. (Have you ever gotten a hypodermic needle from a nurse who is annoyed at the supervisor who won't let her switch shifts?)

If you are able to discuss feelings, bring up these questions: Which feelings are going to be okay to talk about? Are there any feelings that are off-limits? Can we count on each other to be honest with our feelings, or do we need to understand and be able to translate a special signal system? For example, when I am sad, I will let you know by being angry (because I don't do sad well). How about off-limits topics? Can we talk about the finances? The treatments? My promotion? Is anything off-limits? How about sex or my ostomy?

If people don't know the rules, how can they communicate effectively?

Then there is the question of whether it is acceptable for each person involved to do it his or her own way. You see, if you can get others to do everything YOUR way, you do not have to have the anxiety of wondering whether you are doing it okay. Also, you are familiar with your ways, so you feel safest with them. You may even be arrogant enough to think that your way is the right way, even though you and your friends/family are all very different people.

I can recall a family of three young adults whose father was dying. The two daughters were regular visitors, doing all of the traditional things. The son visited less frequently. He found it very difficult to see his father getting weaker. The weaker the father got, the further the son ran. He literally ran, not uncommonly, five miles a day. The father and his daughters seemed to understand. The son had been an athlete, and this was his way of dealing with the feelings that were welling up inside.

Each of us has our own way. It is difficult when someone harshly judges our way or insists that we do it their way. Feeling judged shuts down communication, as does any number of other common difficulties in relating. Watch for these in your situation:

- Your tummy is just a little queasy, so you have decided to take it easy this morning. You don't feel like having orange juice, but you get the third degree from *Directive Dan* about the need for fluids. "What do you mean you don't want your juice? You have to drink it. I will watch while you finish. Now come on." Your brows set, your pulse rushes a little, and you have to decide whether to succumb or to declare your ability to make major decisions, such as whether or not to have four ounces of orange juice. The bottom line is, you don't HAVE to do anything!

- For the sixteenth time today, *Radar Ruth* has said, "You have to rest." You don't feel like resting! This is the first day in the three months since your heart attack that you have enough energy to go out, and she is spoiling your fun. The old rebellious streak is getting fired up. Even though you know it would set you back a week, you are starting to feel like changing a tire, just to let her know who runs your life.

- You are having a lousy day. You just heard your long term disability didn't come through, and now here is *Doting Dotty* with this tray of consommé, apple juice, custard, and cold tea. How are you ever going to get strong enough to go back to work on this stuff? It wouldn't keep a bird alive. So what if you only have half a stomach. You feel like yelling, "Take this crap away and bring me some food!" Better yet, you'd like to throw the tray across the room! In all fairness, you know it isn't the food that is bothering you, and you don't know if you want the embarrassment of watching the cleaning staff be pleasant as they clean it up. And there is no way you are willing to cry!

- *Keen Ken* starts with, "And how are WE today?" He knows the pain of your condition is excruciating. You know you are unable to tolerate it. It has been weeks since you have slept through the night. You have been wondering if life is worth living. You feel too awkward to tell anyone, let alone this insensitive optimist, that you are suicidal, so you say, "Stop this damn pain, or I'm going to put myself out of my misery." You hope someone notices.

- Here comes *Advising Arthur.* He always has it figured out, no matter what the topic is. Yep, there he goes. You don't hear the first part, but the ending is always the same: "Well, it's clear what you have to do." Amazing! You have had the disease ten months, discussed it with him for ten minutes, and he knows what you should do, even though you and umpteen physicians haven't figured it out yet. With luck, he could be bottled and sold at the corner drug store. Even if he proved to be right, you would resent it.

- *Laura Logic* drops by. She is the new surgical resident. She lets you know that the statistics show that surgery is the way to go with your condition. There is a less than six percent fatality rate with this surgery, and the primary surgeon is very skilled. She points out that you are in reasonable health for the operation. What she doesn't seem to understand, partially because you are unwilling to tell anyone, is that you are afraid. Above your neck you are in total agreement. It is the pit in the bottom of your stomach that you are having trouble with. You know that your hesitation comes from remembering that your best friend died of the same surgery, and he was in even better shape than you are. Are you going to tell this lady? No way. You already know she will just tell you more reasons why you need to do this. What you need is someone who will say, "It's okay to be afraid, even if it's illogical."

- *Judging Joyce* is by today. She thinks it is her personal mission in life to shame you into action. She starts in, "You have always been a bit of a wimp. This is a chance to prove to yourself that you have some guts." (Wonder what she says when she wants to get someone discouraged!)

- *Patty Praiser* is the new volunteer in the occupational therapy department. You have gone down for painting this morning just to avoid the boredom of staying in your room, and it's kind of fun to mess around. She is dead serious on being supportive and starts in with, "My, your picture has real potential. I am so glad you came down this morning." Oh boy, here we go. You are color blind, and your four-year-old has more potential! You can tell she is a cousin to Pauline who stopped by the other day and said, "You are coming along fine." Who is she kidding? You are twenty pounds lighter, have to have help walking, and look like Frankenstein on a bad day. If she thinks that's fine, maybe she is sick. How are you supposed to get an accurate picture of how you are doing if people call this "fine"?

- There is always an *Alex the Analyst* around. He is the one who says, "I know why you are being so difficult.

You just want to make your brother feel guilty." Little does he know, you have much more interesting versions of revenge than guilt. But does he stop? NO! He calls in his cousin who specializes, not in your motivations, but in telling you how you feel. She is the one who says, "You're not really angry, you're just tired." You feel like asking her to put down her crystal ball so she can tell you how on earth she knows what you are feeling and thinking. She beats you to it, saying, "I know you would like it if I stayed, but I think I should go. You don't really know what is best for yourself yet." You *do* know you are glad she is leaving. She will be back, though. Are you ready?

● *Sad Sam* is always ready to sympathize. You thought your situation was serious, but by the time he leaves, you are ready to pre-arrange your funeral. He is full of comments like, "I am so sorry this is happening to you. It must be awful. I don't know how you cope." Just what you need, an optimist! Strangely enough, as he leaves he says, "I am sure you'll be fine. Don't you worry." Meanwhile, he has pointed out that you have tubes coming out of every orifice of your body, and that the little line on the monitor is nearly straight!

We all say the wrong things, and do the wrong things, at times. The question is, are you prepared to keep the communication channels open so you can prevent damage to relationships, and when injury occurs, use the communication channels to repair the situation? Will you have realistic expectations of yourself and others during this time of stress?

You may be saying, "I'm no marvel as a communicator." But could you pay a little more attention to expressing and receiving messages about what you and others need? Effective communication is the way by which you will achieve the meeting of your needs. One of the messages you need to convey most clearly is that you care and that you feel cared for.

Illness often does not bring the best out in any of us, particularly if the challenges go on for a long time. Sheer time wears all of us down.

We get tired of being tired. We get frustrated with treatments, and we get concerned about the unknown.

Caregivers wear down with time, too. Many caregivers make the initial mistake of being with the patient day in and day out. Anyone who is with someone day after day, without stopping, starts to get cabin fever. Fatigue, worry, and boredom set in to tell the caregiver that they need a break, too. It is always surprising to a vigilant caregiver who finally goes home for a shower that the patient sleeps soundly while they are gone! How dare the patient! If your caregiver shows signs of cabin fever, you may need to be the one who has to suggest that it's time for a break. Ironic, isn't it: You're the one who is needing the care, and yet you end up taking care of the caregiver! But an illness in your body does not need to mean a deficiency in your capacity to feel and to care for other people.

Cliff was only forty-six when he had a major heart attack. He had been married just a few short and happy weeks. Not long into his intensive care stay, his wife began acting like a nurse rather than the new and cherished wife that she was. Cliff caringly asked how the boys were and was given a patronizing answer that conveyed that he was not to worry about things. A peck on the cheek at the end of visiting hours convinced him he had better speak up right now. He simply told Donna that even though he was lying down, he was still able to give her emotional support; what was wrong with him was in his heart, not his brain. He closed his mini-lecture with, "Don't forget I love you." (She didn't.)

I have temporarily lost all interest in communicating with you. Please stand by.

Ashleigh Brilliant

Getting the Message Across

Communication Strategies

Good communication is advisable at any time, but particularly if you are coping with an illness. There are problems to be solved, decisions to be made, feelings to be dealt with. Remember, it's no time for nonsense. And it is nonsense to believe people can read your mind. Even when you *are* trying to communicate, it may seem impossible to communicate what you really want people to know. Recognize any of these double binds?

- If you talk about symptoms, you're a hypochondriac.

- If you don't talk, you're being too stoic.

- If you stay active, you're denying.

- If you work less, you're just copping out.

- If there is no medical solution, there is no solution.

- If the tests don't show it, you don't have it.

- If you pursue a second opinion, you're "doctor shopping." (Would you stay with a mechanic who couldn't fix your car?)

- If you want to be part of the treatment team, you're demanding and untrusting.

- If you insist on knowing what the medications do, you're difficult.

- If you are well informed, you're compulsive.

- If you are in bed, you can't make decisions for yourself.

- If you are not getting well, you are not trying hard enough.

Sometimes it seems as if you can't win. It is possible to be surrounded by people and still feel as if no one understands. We know there are people who wouldn't understand even if you told them! But, until you tell them, you haven't given them the chance. If you don't consult with anyone, you miss potentially helpful advice. Remember, you don't have to accept the advice, but it is a little risky not even hearing it. If you ask for advice, you might get a totally different perspective.

> Olga had only recently met Karen, but they had developed a trusting relationship quite quickly. They had both come from the old country not long ago. Something was bothering Olga, so she decided she would discuss it with Karen. Olga was short and sweet in her description of the problem: Carl had left the house a year ago to go and get bread. He had never returned. What should she do?
>
> Karen hesitated, then replied, "I t'ink you better go and get the bread yourself."

It is not easy for the people who are trying to understand your situation. If people over-protect you, you may feel smothered and end up feeling resentful and obliged. If people treat you as if you just have the flu, you may feel that they don't recognize the impact this threat is having on your life. If they withdraw, it hurts. If they treat you as you always were, it feels as if they don't recognize you are different. If they treat you differently, it feels as if you have been set apart in some way. Sometimes *they* feel as if they can't win either.

It is not a question whether communication is occurring or not; communication is *always* occurring in some fashion. It is a matter of *what* is being communicated. Most people think of communication as what we say. It is also what we do—and what we do not do—and not only with words. Our bodies talk, too. The next time someone comes through a door, slams it, and stomps through the kitchen, ask them, "What's the matter?" If they reply in stiff terms, "NOTHING!", will you believe them?

Every culture, every family, and every individual has a unique way of communicating. If Uncle Antonio yells, everyone knows he is fine. If Aunt Martha is quiet, something terrible must have happened. If Jack is not socializing, something is bothering him. Each has his or her own personal set of signals in addition to the words that are actually said. The better we know someone, the better we know their message apart from the words.

A young, formerly energetic woman was dying. She was on twenty-four hour oxygen, hardly able to say anything above a whisper. Each day her husband would come over at noon to share lunch with her. He annoyed the attending nurse by telling his wife of the progress on the back deck, the efforts on the garden, and the preparations for their up-coming camping trip. The nurse left the room, frustrated with the husband's inappropriate topics of conversation, and returned later, assuming she would provide the support seemingly absent from the husband. She asked the patient, "How do you feel about Bob's plans for the summer?"

The young woman's face radiated. She replied, "Isn't he wonderful? He comes in every day to cheer me up. We both know I will never be going camping."

Little did the young woman know what an important lesson she had just taught one humbled nurse.

An older couple requested to talk with counseling services. Every week each of them would wait while the other talked to the counselor. They flatly refused to have even one session together. They spoke highly of each other, but admitted that they had never talked about difficult things together. They had just gone about doing what needed to be done, and this strategy had always worked for them. They were not about to start a whole new way of relating at this point, although they were each very supportive of the other getting counseling.

At one point the husband, Adam, did want to tell his dying wife how important she was to him and how much he had appreciated how she had supported him through tough times in the years past. He wrote her a long and beautiful letter which she carried with her literally at all times until her death. Their communication, puzzling to an outsider, was perfectly understood by each other.

Effective communication is a matter of getting your *intended* message across. We are not recommending *how* you should communicate. We would, however, like to emphasize the importance of being aware of doing so, and provide some suggestions.

"There is a time and a place" is an expression that applies to communicating. If you have something important you want to discuss with a friend, a physician, or a family member keep in mind these three guidelines:

● **Pick the Time**
During illness you may find you are more impulsive and that your feelings are closer to the surface. This makes your timing somewhat off balance at times. Things spill out that you were not planning. The time to announce to your family that you are going into life-threatening surgery is not just as you are getting onto the stretcher. The time to demand that your teenager clean her room is just not as she goes off to her final exams. Any time, however, is a good time to say, "I care."

● **Pick the Place**
A dinner party is not the setting at which to announce you just had a rectal exam (unless, of course, you have a good sense of humor and you don't want to come to another dinner party). The place to discuss your will with your lawyer is not in the middle of an eight-bed unit. (Make arrangements with the head nurse in advance to use a consulting room. If the nurse balks, which is not likely, ask to speak to an administrator.) You have a right to some privacy and dignity. Don't grovel in order to have a few minutes of discussion with someone who is influencing your health, or your life.

● **Pick the Person**
There is little point in trying to dent a mountain with a toothpick. Select with some thought what you want to say to whom. Some people are great for laughs, some for help with practical things in life, some for listening to what you are feeling inside. If you pick the comic to tell your feelings to, you will feel as bad as he or she feels awkward. If you pick the empathizer for helping with practical things, you may just keep hearing, "Oh, Sally, I am so sorry this is happening to you," when what

> you really want is someone to feed the cats. If you are looking for someone to cry with, don't expect it will be Mr. Logical. He will just ruin a good cry explaining it away.

In our experience there are also three main targets for effective communication:

- yourself;

- your healthcare team;

- others who care for you.

COMMUNICATING WITH YOURSELF

This is not as strange as it sounds; you do it all the time. Your body is constantly communicating with you. It tells you when you hurt, when you are hungry, and when you are tired. Now that's not so strange, is it? Every time you are thinking something over in your head, you are communicating with yourself.

Children have the good sense to lie down and go to sleep when they are tired. It doesn't matter where they are. If they are feeling lonely, they will crawl up on someone's lap or ask for a hug. We are not recommending that you crawl up on someone's lap, but we are suggesting that you spend time with yourself. Actually carry on a conversation with yourself. (If you do it out loud, close the door or they will send the people in white coats and put you on medication that makes your head go funny!)

One rather well-known, old Greek philosopher put it this way: "Know Thy Self."

No one knows you better than you do. You have had to live with your quirks longer than anyone else. If you have discussions with yourself, you will not find any ghosts in the closet that you didn't already know were there, but you might chase a few of them away.

Some people use an "Inner Guide." They ask themselves a question and then wait quietly for an answer. They begin to understand that there is a part of themselves that is wise and can guide them through this difficult time if they will just stop and get to know that side of themselves.

Others use their imagination and visualize situations that they have or will encounter. They practice new ways of doing things in their minds, much as they would learn lines for a play. One fellow described being ill as feeling as if he was the main actor who didn't know his lines.

Others find a journal very helpful. Some keep a very organized journal and have one section for their concerns and practical problems, one for dreams, one for feelings, one for conversations they hope to have, and so forth. By getting things on paper they often feel relief at clearing their minds and are amazed that a solution often emerges that they never thought of before. (Some people hate writing. If you are one of them, a journal isn't your best move.)

Whether you are going to gaze at your ceiling or write in your journal, here are some starter questions to ask yourself.

- What do I expect of myself?

- What am I feeling?

- What am I thinking about illness, sex, friends, work, etc.?

- What part of what I am thinking do I want to communicate?

- How well am I communicating with others?

- How am I judging myself and others?

The whole idea is that, if you are communicating with yourself, your ideas are clearer, and, if your ideas are clearer, you can communicate with your healthcare team and loved ones more readily, not to mention your unloved ones.

COMMUNICATING WITH YOUR HEALTHCARE TEAM

Everyone knows that a good doctor-patient relationship is important. Notice that we didn't say, "a good doctor." We said, "a good *relationship*." Doctors vary in their skills and in their bedside manners. So do patients. The difficulty comes when the personalities of patient and doctor are incompatible. Much like any other partnership, there has to be minimal communication for the relationship to be tolerable, and most people want the relationship with their doctors to be mutually trusting and responsible. The two most common traits we look for in a physician are competency and compassion. They can come in four combinations: competency with compassion, competency without compassion, incompetency with compassion, or incompetency without compassion.

Each of us would prefer the first combination. However, in medical school only a few hours of doctors' training are spent on how to relate to patients. Doctors also are not immune to having quirks in their personalities, and certainly they have their share of hassles in the day. Nor are they immune to being insensitive because of their personalities or their training. Some are plain intolerant of patients who are looking for a partnership rather than obedience-training. Others welcome patients who are willing to share the responsibility for their recoveries.

What are your attitudes toward physicians? How are you going to find a doctor with whom you can work, and vice versa? What are your expectations of your doctor? Have you talked to him or her about your expectations, or are you just waiting until your doctor doesn't meet them? How heavily are you relying on your doctor for a sense of caring? How likely is your doctor to express his or her caring, given your doctor's personality?

Here are some hints about talking with physicians:

- Be sure you know who is responsible for you. Where does the buck stop? It is great having a "team" but clarify who is *your* doctor.

- Forget trying to read doctors' expressions. Most of them went to poker school.

- Tell your doctor how you want to be treated. How much information do you want or not want?

- Know your bottom line. What is non-negotiable? Remember that it can change when the circumstances change.

- If your doctor recommends any of those wonder drugs, *wonder* what they are and how to use them. Ask questions! We know a woman who swallowed her suppositories and reported that they didn't work!

- Your responsibility is to report symptoms. Let your doctor know what you are experiencing. You are not playing fair if you delay reporting your symptoms.

- If you don't feel you are getting answers, just keep asking.

- At the end of a discussion, ask for a summary or give one. Simply say, "It seems what we have discussed is. . ." If you have misunderstood something, this gives your physician a chance to correct it. This goes for discussions with your other healthcare professionals as well.

- Delegate someone you trust to be your advocate and spokesperson in the healthcare world.

- Make friends with the receptionist in your physician's office.

- Have a good general practitioner with whom you can talk, someone who knows the overall story and who knows you.

- If you are satisfied with the service you are getting, write a letter to administration.

- If you are dissatisfied, let your physician know. If the situation seems to continue, write an administrator or switch physicians. Do something!

- Use expressions that improve communication, like:
    Could you explain further?
    I am not comfortable with. . .
    I am puzzled about. . .
    What can I expect from. . .?
    What do I do if this doesn't work?
    How long should I tolerate any side effects?
    When should I see you next?

Your physician is your partner in your effort to get well. Like you, he or she is an individual and will have his or her own ways of communicating, some effective, some less so. Although training for doctors does not necessarily prepare them to be good at talking or listening, most do care, even if they are not good at saying so. Some are excellent communicators. With others, you may need to provide the leadership.

Also keep in mind that doctors are not personally responsible for *everything* that happens to you during your illness. Many things are the result of the medical systems in which you are getting care. Clinics and hospitals almost have a personality of their own. You can sense it from their color, from the pace at which people move, from the waiting rooms. In all kinds of different ways, they can send helpful or unhelpful messages, such as:

- We care about you, but don't get sick after 4:30.

- We control your time.

- Your time is less important than ours.

- You are a child. We will tell you what to wear and when to turn the lights out.

- "You won't throw up" (but they leave a kidney dish).

- "This won't hurt" (but it does).

- The whole place seems to say, "Don't laugh!"

Time is always an issue. Nothing ever seems to happen quickly enough. We suggest that, in a hospital, you assume you are on another planet. Take earth time and multiply by 1.5 to get hospital time. Your other choice is to be very frustrated by what you feel are delays. And they may be! They might also be legitimate in that the treatment is dependent on some test results which are delayed, and so forth. Things could always be better, but what is wrong is often not because of any specific person. If you really want to help make things different, ask one of your healthcare team to recommend someone to whom you could talk or write. Or check to see if your hospital has a patient representative whom you could contact. There are other alternatives. Try some of these while you wait:

- Plan the revolution you will lead when you get well.

- Write and market a poster "101 Things To Do While You Wait."

- Read humor books.

- Bring your knitting.

- Pick your teeth.

- Plan a vacation.

- Write a letter.

- Write a poem.

- Talk to a volunteer.

- Do a research project on whether people with brown eyes get attended to first.

- Organize a sing-along.

- Bring along a book on patient rights. It makes them nervous.

Flexibility is also an issue. Some systems seem to take the patient into less account than others. A hard driving, tough truck driver found his stay in a palliative care unit difficult. He saw no reason why he should turn the light out in his private room at ten o'clock. Finally, he declared, "Look, the lights are going to go out for good, soon enough. I am not turning them off at ten just because you want to tuck me in."

Other units may be much more flexible, like the unit that arranged for the security guard and the head nurse to be elsewhere so that a favorite collie could be smuggled up the back stairs to spend a few precious moments with his master.

COMMUNICATING WITH OTHERS

Living with other people involves having a contract with them. It is not necessarily formal, but just think about your day. You usually know who does what and when. Some contracts are more flexible than others. If you live or work with another person, you have a contract of some sort that you may need to renegotiate during illness. Who is responsible for what? Who will decide what? Who is going to have what information and how are they going to get it?

Remember, it's not only *what* you say but *how* you say things that makes a difference in how people hear you. Just try saying, 'I never said he dated Alice," putting the emphasis on a different word each time. See what we mean? The same is true even if words are not used.

Jocelyn's family sent a mixed message when they all came to send her off to major surgery in another state. But they didn't have a thing to say to the previously robust athlete who was now just over eighty pounds and fading fast. Their silence spoke loudly when they all lined up for one last somber picture as a family. (By the way, Jocelyn lived, and she kids them now about the family portrait technique!)

If you and the person or persons you are living with enjoy writing, a dialogue journal can be very helpful. You or they can write beefs and/or bouquets to each other. If you want a response, agree on a signal. (In our family, you have to write back if the pen is in the journal.)

Learn the value of good questions. "Why" is not all that useful: "Why are you sad?" Sometimes, you just don't have an answer. It is more useful to ask open-ended expressions like:

- What does that feel like?

- Can you say more about that?

- How are you feeling about it now?

- What does that mean for you?

- How would you like things to be?

- I am wondering if. . .

Notice all of the questions invite more than a "Yes" or a "No" answer.

Practice using "feeling" words: "I feel [*mad, glad, bad, sad*]." When you are good at those, go on to the next level, using gradations of the basic feeling words: "I feel [*annoyed, frustrated, angry, furious*]" or "[*disappointed, down, hurt, sad, depressed*]."

Notice that the words "I feel" precede the feeling word. This is a way of owning your feelings. As you practice using this phrase, you'll get used to it. Yes, we know your grandmother doesn't approve of being self-centered. Well, in this case, your grandmother is wrong, even though she makes great ginger cookies.

Owning your feelings is a crucial step in maintaining healthy communication and healthy relationships. Notice the difference between saying, "I am disappointed in you for not cleaning the garage," and "You lousy brat! I told you to clean the garage." Judging people does not get things to change as often as respect does. It is hard for the receiver to empathize with you if you are yelling at them. All they want to do is get away or retaliate and even if, out of fear, they do clean the garage, no one gets to feel good about it.

There could be a whole book just on communication. (Reading this chapter probably felt as if there was.) For the next few days, listen to your own communication. Maybe there is something you could be doing to make communication even more constructive. Never mind what *they* could do. It's only *you* who can change *you*.

The song of a nightingale is more enticing than that of a crow.

Ronna Fay Jevne

The Ignorant and the Unwashed

Handling the Unhelpful

Some people, even well-meaning and well-educated persons, can be incredibly insensitive when it comes to seriously ill patients.

Every seriously ill person is inundated with a torrent of advice from presumably well-meaning friends and relatives. It seems that everyone has either obtained a night-school diploma in medicine or is an internationally recognized authority on your particular problem. At a minimum, most of them know three or four people with your exact type of illness who would be alive today if only they had heeded the particular type of advice that is being bestowed on you!

You'll probably also encounter people who feel that it is inappropriate for you to make decisions about your own treatment — they feel all decisions should be left to the professionals caring for you. Their advice is to allow doctors to handle everything. After all, doctors know what they are doing. And it is heretical to question authority.

How can you handle the problem of too much advice? First, make sure that you have absolute confidence in the individuals caring for you. Make sure that they are all properly credentialed or Board-Certified. Ask other patients and health professionals what they think of them. Second, make sure you fully understand the diagnosis, prognosis, and treatment being suggested. If your doctor cannot explain these to you, see someone who can. Get a second or third opinion if you think it is appropriate.

In any event, make sure that you feel everything that should be done has been done with regard to your illness. Once this has been accomplished, you'll be in a much better position to deal with the advice of others.

Let's also be fair. Many of the people who make a variety of alternative care suggestions are genuinely trying to help. Many of them are also trying to deal with their own anxieties about your illness. After all, if you can have this illness, so can they!

As you already may have experienced, you can often tell what people are thinking, but not saying, by the way they greet you. It usually begins with a "How *aaarre* you," accompanied by a furrowed brow and solicitous look. What they may really be thinking is, "It makes me anxious to see you around. Why don't you drop dead and get it over with?"

An appropriate response might be to tell them that you appreciate their concern, but that you just pooped in your pants and you're rushing home to change them. Ask them if they'd like to come by and help with the laundry later. If you get a taker, you know you have a real friend and you might share the truth with them.

Let them know that, instead of asking how you are, they might give you a big hug, tell you how glad they are to see you and how much they care about you! Tell them also that you've already heard about Uncle Sylvester who had the exact same type of cancer you have and who died right after they opened him up and let the air get to it, thereby causing it to spread all over his body. (Particularly because yours is ovarian, and you doubt that Uncle Sylvester was in need of a sex change operation!)

An alternative is to respond like the Irish priest who awoke one day to find a dead donkey on the parish house lawn. He proceeded to call the local police station and said, "Good morning, this is Father Murphy."

"Ah yes, Father, and what can I do for you today?" responded the policeman.

"There's a dead jackass on the parish house lawn!" said the Father.

There was a brief pause and the policeman said, "I thought it was the responsibility of the Church to bury the dead."

Father Murphy was taken aback by this less-than-helpful reply but quickly responded, " 'Tis true, 'tis true, but it's also the responsibility of the Church to notify the next of kin!"

If you run into any people who seriously want to be supportive or helpful but don't know how, suggest that they begin by telling you about formerly seriously ill patients who are cured and doing well, rather than about other patients who are doing poorly. If you have cancer, remind them that half of all cancer patients are cured. If even one person has ever recovered from your illness, why can't you? Ask them to support you in your effort to be that person!

Know how to become closer to them and make them an even better friend? ASK THEM FOR A FAVOR! It doesn't matter what; just ask them to do something for you. Asking is the best way to consolidate a friendship. It sounds paradoxical, doesn't it? But it works! You're telling them, "You have something or some skill that I value; please share it with me." And wouldn't some ripe tomatoes from their garden taste good right now?

Serious illness scares people. It probably dates back to the days of the black plague when contagion was spread by person-to-person contact. Let people know that cancer or other serious illness, especially AIDS, is not transmitted by touching. They can touch you without concern. That applies to friends, strangers, and intimate associates as well.

When appropriate, refer them to the literature on recovery from serious illness and ask them to help you find additional inspirational reading. Some suitable books might be *Anatomy of an Illness* by Norman Cousins; *The Cancer Survivors — and How They Did It* by Judith Glassman; *The Healer Within* by Stephen Locke; *Superimmunity* by Paul Pearsall; and *We, the Victors* by Curtis Bill Pepper.[1]

If all else fails, avoid going to places where you're likely to run into people you would rather not see. Similarly, cultivate the acquaintance of persons who have surmounted their illness and find out how they did it.

Last and best of all, GET WELL and show everyone that it can be done! Then once you've gotten well, tell everyone about it and how you did it. Most of what we've just discussed involves assertive communication skills and, by sheer coincidence, that's what the next chapter is all about!

---

[1] Refer to the Bibliography for information on these and other additional recommended readings.

I've just learnt about his illness; let's hope it's nothing trivial.

Irvin Cobb

You're Sitting on My Hat

Asserting Yourself

Few of us would fail to tell someone that they're sitting on our hat. But many of us fail to speak up when other injuries occur. We all secretly admire the restaurant patron who refuses to take the table in front of the kitchen door when others are available. But not all of us would speak up under similar circumstances.

Well? Is your life worth fighting for or not? Of course it is! We've already talked about everyone's expectations that you're going to be ready for the wheelchair, nursing home, or funeral parlor any minute now. Well, THEY'RE WRONG!! Don't just sit there. Tell them so! And, better yet, prove it to them by getting better. Better yet, get well!!

What's worth being assertive about? What's *not*? People can push you around about some things, but not:

- that you be fully informed about your illness;

- that you participate in all decision-making;

- that your symptoms are evaluated fully and to your satisfaction;

- that you need to trust all the people who are caring for you;

- that you will not wait unreasonable lengths of time for anything important;

- that you will be listened to — fully.

STRATEGIES IN THE DOCTOR'S OFFICE

Earlier we suggested bringing a tape recorder and a friend to the doctor's office so you can remember what the doctor says. If you want to be even more assertive, a court reporter might get your doctor's attention.

Here's some more things you might try:

- Bring a list of questions. Check them off as they are answered.

- Give your doctor a grade before you leave.

- Teach your doctor how to print. (The nurses and pharmacist will thank you.)

- Ask to read your chart. After all, you paid for it.

- Sit between your doctor and the door.

- Bring M & M's and feed them to your doctor.

- If your doctor doesn't take the time to talk to you, grab some article of your doctor's clothing and hold on until your questions get answered. We're reluctant to recommend you literally grab his or her necktie, but we do suggest you do something to grab your doctor's attention.

STRATEGIES IN THE HOSPITAL

- Find out who's in charge.

- Know your patient rights.

- Bring your own sheets, bathrobe, and soap.

- Take down any pictures in the room you don't like and replace them with ones you do like.

- Send back the food if it's cold. If necessary, threaten to bring in your own microwave.

- If a staff person is annoying you, talk to his or her

supervisor. If that gets no action, consider contacting the patient advocate or the local TV station investigative reporter.

- Never wear a hospital gown when street clothes will do.

- Never take off your underwear except to change it.

- Play hooky. All hospitals let patients out on pass. Save them the paperwork.

- Don't take any medicines unless you know what they're for and how soon they're supposed to work and when you can stop them.

- Accept nothing on faith unless it feels good to do so.

STRATEGIES FOR LIVING

What is the difference between assertiveness and absurdity? We're not sure anymore. We recommend "absurdiveness" training. Do one outrageous thing every day. Stand up and demand your rights! You are entitled to the right of life, liberty, and freedom from pain. How about . . .

- ordering a pizza right now?

- sending a strip-o-gram to the widower down the block?

- kissing your dog? (If you don't have one, borrow the neighbor's.)

- buying donuts? (If you're a diabetic, give them to the first child you see after leaving the store.)

- getting yourself a pair of lacy black underpants and wearing them in the doctor's office?

- writing "BOO" over your navel and waiting for the doctor to find it?

Always, always, have pictures of your grandchildren, children, dogs, cats, boats, garden, or even your newly redecorated bathroom and show them to everyone twice! And then quiz them about it. If they don't pass, make them look at all of your pictures again.

THE ONLY ENEMY IS SILENCE!

WHAT DID YOU SAY? SPEAK UP. WE CAN'T HEAR YOU!

Were you trying to say "No"? That's the hardest word in the English language to say. We'll give you some tips. When someone asks something of you, or tells you do to something, you can say "No." You don't have to plead inadequacy, or be angry, guilty, or apologetic.

The key to saying NO begins with assessing the request in terms of your own goals. Ask yourself, "Do I want to do this? Who am I trying to please? Do I have the resources (time, energy, money, motivation)?" This is the wrong time in your life to try to win the congeniality award. If you need more information, ask for it. Then give yourself a bit of time to decide. If your answer is NO, rehearse how you will say it. Practice over and over until your statement is free of anger, apology, or excuses. A short, quick statement is all that is needed.

 A thick skin is a gift from God.

Konrad Adenauer

SECTION 5

FEELINGS

Getting Off the Roller Coaster

Am I Normal?

Understanding Your Feelings

"Am I normal? Do other people feel this way?" These are the questions people most frequently ask. Think for a moment. If the answer is, "Yes, you are normal," are you better off? Normal isn't necessarily healthy! In some situations the normal thing to do is to die!

Think of the people you know whom you really enjoy. Would you say, "I really like or admire them because they're so normal"?

How about your epitaph: "Here lies _____. She was normal."

Ever hear a little kid say, "When I grow up, I want to be normal"?

Why even consider *normal* as something to which you'd want to aspire? However, you *are* normal if you are one of the many who need reassurance that they are normal. A common conversation in my office goes like this:

Patient: Doc, I don't know what's wrong with me. I was doing just fine. The kids are settling down. The finances are in order. My long term disability has finally come through, but I just can't get used to this idea of dying.

Doctor: Have you ever done this before?

Patient: What do you mean?

Doctor: I mean, have you ever known before that you were ill enough that you were expected to die?

Patient: Well, no.

Doctor: What do you expect of yourself as you are going through this?

Patient: What do you mean? I was doing fine until recently. I wasn't crying or anything. Suddenly, it feels different. I feel so much. I don't know what's happening to me.

Doctor: So, you figured you'd get a terminal diagnosis, do all the arranging of life affairs that is logical under the circumstances, keep saying pleasant things to people who look at you as if you were already dead, have invasive treatments, throw up most of your meals, know that you have likely had your last birthday, and you are wondering why you are having some feelings?

Patient: I never thought of it that way. You mean my feelings are normal?

Doctor: Yes, they're normal.

Patient: Thanks, Doc, I feel better.

What people are really asking is, "Is there something wrong with me? Am I going crazy or can this be normal? How similar or different are my experiences from those of other people who are going through the same thing?"

The problem is that you are not like anyone else, and what you are going through is not the same as it is for anyone else.

For example, you could be unfortunate enough to be one of two people who fall into the same crocodile-infested river. There are always different factors that influence who survives. How deep is the part of the river in which you fall? Can you swim? Are you armed? Are the crocodiles sleepy or hungry? Do you have a buddy to help you into the boat again? Do you owe the buddy a large sum of money? Does this happen when you are twenty or sixty-five? Have you any experience in these waters?

The point is, what is normal for one person is not normal for another. We are raised in different families. We have different successes and failures. We have different resources, support, and skills. We think differently. Why should we all have similar — translate, NORMAL — experiences? You have to decide what is normal for you.

What is the toughest situation you have ever faced? How did you get through it? How tough is your situation now compared to that one? You have known yourself longer than anyone else has. It is YOU who must decide what is normal for you.

We each have our own strengths, our own quirks, our own limits. Some people seem invincible. Some are more vulnerable. "Normal" has as many variations as there are people!

One young man arrived at the hospital to see his mother a couple of days after her surgery. When she couldn't be found, a nurse reported to him that his mother had been asked to start walking. She had resented the request because she had considerable post-surgical pain. When pushed, she had finally said, "Fine, I will run." She had last been seen doing a hasty shuffle toward pediatrics.

The nurse was concerned that the son would be distressed. He simply smiled and said, "You don't know my mother!"

The nurses got to know more of this side of his mother later, when she had some difficulty with eating. Without consulting the patient, a nurse arrived with an intravenous, announcing this would be supper. The patient wanted to know why. The answer was, "The doctor ordered it." The patient demanded that a doctor appear before 4:30 p.m. or else she would eat a huge meal. At 5:00 p.m. she went to the hospital cafeteria and down went the pork chops, gravy, mashed potatoes, corn, and a piece of pie. At 5:30 p.m. a doctor did arrive. The patient announced that a heavy meal seemed to be just what she had needed.

Her behavior was perhaps not normal by some standards. She did, however, have character! And today she is well and still running her life. What she was doing was normal and healthy for her.

People tend to think anything *new* is somehow not normal. But illness is a time when you may learn about new sides of yourself that you had not even known existed before. If you are a perpetual optimist, you may find it disconcerting when you have that well-earned "down day." If you are a weary pessimist, you may be surprised to discover that your illness draws from you a strength you never knew you had. Give yourself a chance!

The range of NORMAL is very broad. Yes, you are normal if you feel a sense of loss, if you feel a sense of challenge, if you feel cheated, or if you feel appreciative of the life you have had so far.

Illness has often been discussed in terms of the number of losses you may experience: The loss of predictability; the loss of status; the loss of body image; the loss of your role as a parent, partner, or friend. Feelings associated with loss vary, and you may have any or all of them, in almost any order. You are normal if:

- you find yourself denying the diagnosis or prognosis;

- you find yourself in a state of facing facts and fighting facts;

- you resent being ill (after all, it has turned your life upside down);

- you get discouraged;

- you want more time;

- you break into tears unexpectedly;

- you want to yell, "No! You don't understand!"

You are also normal if you *don't* have a whole well of overwhelming feelings. There are people who are actually relieved to find out they are sick. They may be comforted to realize that what they were afraid were signs of laziness or depression are really signs of unwellness. There are people who say illness is the best thing that ever happened to them. That can be a normal reaction, particularly if someone's circumstances are such that they previously have been throwing away their lives.

What is normal is very dependent on the whole picture. How old are you? How experienced are you with fighting for your life? Who is around to help? How serious is your illness? How satisfied were you with life before your illness? These all influence how painful the experience of illness is — not just how physically painful, but how emotionally painful.

When you are hurt physically, pain in your body warns you that something is wrong. When you hurt emotionally, your feelings are the pain indicators. They tell you what kind of emotional injury you have incurred. By listening to your feelings, you can begin to understand something about how to deal with the pain and heal from the injury.

When things are going right, your feelings may be positive. When you are having a sense of loss, you may feel sad. When you are annoyed at someone, you may have a feeling of anger. If you are scared, fear or anxiety arrives. Even a small child can tell if a person is sad or angry. The confusion comes if you have been raised in a family where tears were not allowed, so you had to yell whenever you felt sad.

Any strong feeling that you don't like is just a signal that you need to do something different. The standard view is that you have to talk about your feelings, but that is not as easy as it sounds.

What is normal in terms of talking about feelings varies a great deal. Not all of us are aware of our feelings and still others of us are not willing to talk about our feelings with others, particularly strangers. Different cultures have different ways of expressing feelings, too. Not everyone has to talk everything out. In some cultures and families, things are done on a more nonverbal level. That can be very normal, if it is part of your upbringing. Why should you belong to the "Tell Everything Club" just because you are sick?

If you are a private person, it is nonsense for people to think that you will suddenly become a person who is going to share your feelings with every well-intentioned inquirer who feels you should now trust them as your confidante. Many people find it difficult to talk about their feelings, even if something is bothering them.

I recall being asked to see a woman receiving treatment in the day program. The doctor and the nurses were worried about her, and she reluctantly agreed to talk to someone from counseling services. I used my best bedside manner and got nowhere. Because I believe it is everyone's right to do things their way, I finally decided that to probe further would feel like one more intrusive treatment to her. I closed by saying, "I have asked you a number of questions. Have you anything you would like to ask me?"

She was pleasant and said, "No, I don't think so. I just saw you so I could get the doctors and nurses off my back."

I wished her well and started for the door. She called me back and said, "Maybe I do have a question. I think I'm doing okay, but when do the nightmares go away?"

Stop asking the question, "Am I normal?" and start asking, "Is this helping? Am I thinking, feeling, and doing things that will help me in the long run?" Changing the way you think, the way you express your feelings, and the way you do things can seem foreign and awkward initially. Feeling different does not have to be a problem. It can be an adventure!

Survivors are normal people who decide to make remarkable choices.

Ronna Fay Jevne

Getting Off the Roller Coaster

Changing Your Feelings

Remember your first roller coaster ride? Did you go reluctantly or were you exhilarated by what you were about to do? Did you ride with your eyes open or closed? Did you scream or freeze in silence? When it was over, did you decide it was your parents' way of getting even for all the times you had left the peanut butter out, or were you so thrilled you were ready to go again?

Illness is a lot like a first roller coaster ride. It can generate all kinds of feelings. If you are lucky, your ride may only be a ferris wheel version. A ferris wheel still has ups and downs and gives the feeling of being out of control, but it goes a little slower and stops more often.

When serious illness strikes, your world can be turned upside down. There are adjustments after adjustments, unknowns after unknowns, decisions after decisions, problems after problems. It is no wonder life feels as if you were riding a roller coaster controlled by a kamikaze pilot. However, the roller coaster does have a remote control. You can take charge of your ride.

One youngster discovered it was possible to have control even on his first ferris wheel ride. When it stopped at the top to begin the unloading process below, five-year-old Will decided he had had enough of sitting beside a perfect stranger and was getting out. He loudly insisted that the ferris wheel start down right that moment or he was jumping. The incident created considerable flurry below. In seconds the ferris wheel was moving again.

Some people don't believe they can take charge of anything, let alone their own lives. Well, sorry, folks. What you *have* been is what you have been. What you are *going to be* is still up for grabs. As a matter of fact, illness can be the very thing you have been looking for in order to make a few changes in your life you might not have had the guts to make before.

Take Ted for instance. He was an ex-cop of seventeen years, turned teacher and school principal. He was a little overweight, a workaholic, and unhappily married. He was Mr. Upstanding Citizen, president of this, coordinator of that, taking courses toward his graduate degree, a foster parent, politically active. At forty-six he had his first major heart attack right in his office. When relatives he hadn't seen for years started parading past his intensive care bed, he gave things a second thought. Later, he also sought out professional help. He wanted life to be different, but he wasn't sure how to start. But start he did. Difficult as the choices were, he chose resignation from his principalship, divorce from his wife, commitment to cardiac rehabilitation. He embarked on a lifestyle of not only survival, but of well-being. Ten years later, he is still teaching, happily remarried, and treasuring each day.

Young Mac was devastated when, at nineteen, he got testicular cancer. With the weight loss and the chemotherapy, his handsome young body was unrecognizable in a few months. His friends disappeared. His world was transformed. He had never been so scared in his life. His macho mask didn't hold. At twenty-two, he now says, "Illness was the best thing that ever happened to me. Before, I was wasting my life. Now, I have goals."

Diane was forty when she had her mastectomy. It didn't help when her husband chose that particular time in their lives to have an affair. She wasn't sure if she was more angry or more hurt. They had had everything. A beautiful home, two clever children in boarding school, no worries. But it looked like her world was going to disappear. The road was tough. She decided the marriage was worth saving, but that she had lost some of the spunk her husband had married her for and that a number of things about their family life needed to change. Several years later, she is running her own business. Her husband, Lawrence, is making the occasional meal, and the children are attending school at home. Needless to say, some changes occurred. They began with Diane.

Where do you start? You start with a willingness and you start with yourself. Since you are the only person over whom you really have control, trying to get others to change just uses up precious energy. You don't have to know how you are going to do it, but you do have to be willing to believe that SOMEHOW your life can be different. The

1970's poster, "THIS IS THE FIRST DAY OF THE REST OF YOUR LIFE," is true. You don't have to like it, but you'd be smart to believe it! The first person with whom you have to be honest is YOU. You can only change what you are willing to notice. If, of course, you don't notice that you are being a monster or that you are falling apart, then you probably won't change anything.

Helga was referred to me by the Pain Control Team. They were unable to control her hip pain. In hobbled a large European woman. Her accent was strong and her character even more so. When I asked her about her pain, she talked not about her hip, but about her anger toward her husband. She had been expected to die several years previously, so when they moved to a new city, she decorated the apartment in what she considered to be masculine color tones, with the thought that they would be appropriate when she was gone. Then her husband up and died! (Not deliberately I am sure, as their marriage, by all reports was a very satisfying one to both of them).

She was left alone with no caregiver to accompany her through her illness. Suddenly her sons could do nothing right! They married the wrong girls, asked to borrow money too often, and didn't visit often enough. The church was too rigid, and she hated being told that a "real Christian" wouldn't smoke! (Who wouldn't hate being told what not to do?)

She baked relentlessly but resented it when people would invite her to a social function and suggest that she bring one of her special cakes. She, of course, informed no one of her specific resentments. She simply grew more and more angry and puzzled that fewer and fewer people would visit. She described her situation with a tone of judgment that would have made a hangman cringe. I timidly suggested to her that, were her chair not between me and the door, I might be as tempted as those in her world to withdraw from her. She promised to think about how others might be experiencing her.

Somewhat to my surprise, she returned a week later. She had traded her walker for two canes. She plunked herself down, drove one cane into the new rug I had just spent a year pleading for (and which still bears the autograph of that day), and announced in a loud voice, "I have been such a beetch! Why didn't someone tell me? Thank you so much for telling me. I apologized to six people this week."

After repairing a number of relationships that had become strained with her unexpressed grief, Helga began life as a single person. She now walks using one cane. Her first step was her willingness to change and to start with herself.

Being honest with yourself is not easy. Try it. What are you keeping secret? What don't you like to admit, even to yourself? What are you scared to give up? Your image? The illusion that you control everything? The idea that you are helpless and have to be taken care of? We've all got something we don't want to change. What's yours?

After the willingness to change, what then? Take a couple of days off. You have earned it. Just enjoy knowing you are going to change something. (If you are compulsive, you can immediately start figuring out what you want instead of what is going on now.) Don't waste a lot of time berating yourself for not starting sooner in life. It's a waste of time, too, to whine and worry about how inadequate you are, and how you might fall short of the goals you set. Come on, I challenge you. Name me one thing that got better because you worried about it. If anything gets better, it is because someone did something about it. You don't have to talk a lot about what you are going to do differently either. What's the saying? . . . "When all is said and done, too much is said and too little done."

You don't get where you want to go by worrying or talking about all your faults. Becoming aware and acknowledging your faults to yourself, and sometimes to others, is a first step. For example, Helga had to admit to herself she had been acting like "a beetch." She was then able to take action to start healing and developing the relation-ships she wanted. We get where we want to go on our *strengths*, not our faults. Everyone has at least one strength. That's all you need. Let's go.

Sure, you may falter. Who doesn't? When we are learning something new, we are much like a child. We don't say (or I hope we don't say) to children when they stumble as they are learning to walk, "You dummy, you are supposed to do this perfectly the first time! You sure are an inadequate kid." So the first or even the second time that you are fighting a life-threatening illness, don't say to yourself, "I sure am stupid." You can't be everything to everyone all the time when, at the same time, you are learning a whole new life style. Save the humbleness and the apologies for when you are well. You can't afford the energy right now.

A number of patients hang up reminders on their refrigerators, on their bathroom mirrors, wherever they will notice them often, posters that say, "I do not have to apologize for being ill." Make your own poster with whatever you need to encourage yourself. Here are some suggestions:

- Rome wasn't built in a day. I can take time to get well.
- I will make choices for health today.
- Have I laughed today?
- Have I hugged a friend today?

Build in the encouragement you need. If you have family or friends whom you trust, ask them how they think you are handling things and what they think you need. Consider their answers, but don't take their words as truth. Remember, they may have their own hangups and could unknowingly be dumping them on your emotional field. It's your life. You have to decide what you want and what you are willing to do. Negotiation is fine, but the bottom line is, if you give away responsibility for your life, don't be surprised if you don't like someone else's management style.

Being responsible for your life includes being responsible for what you are feeling. This is one of three tough lessons in life, which, once learned, make life a little easier to tolerate:

- Life isn't fair.
- People aren't always reasonable.
- You are responsible for your own feelings.

If you believe someone else can *make* you feel, you are constantly vulnerable. Think about these statements:

- "You make me angry."
- "You are driving me crazy."
- "You hurt me."

Even though we hear phrases like these all the time, that doesn't make them correct. No one can *make* us feel any particular way.

Think about it. If you were the third car back from a stop light and you moved ahead when the light changed, but the car ahead of you didn't, how would you feel as you heard the sound of the bumpers introducing each other? Some people would be angry that the other person wasn't watching. Some embarrassed. Others guilty. Someone else might be afraid that the 6'4" guy in the car ahead was going to be very unfriendly. Still others would feel relieved that no one was hurt. If someone else can *make* you feel, how come there can be such a variation in response to one situation?

That is not to say that we live in total isolation, but we do have choices. Anyone who has ever lived with a teenager, and survived, knows that there are choices as to how to react. The picnics in the family room can be simply a training ground for tidiness or a source of anger. The mood swings can be antagonizing or they can be seen as a young adult dealing with an overdose of hormones. Watching teenagers go through an emotional roller coaster is bad enough. We don't have to join them.

Other situations are no different. There is often an immediate reaction that seems to be so automatic it is out of our control. That's just habit. Even that can change with time. We do have choices about how we want to feel. It might take a bit of talking to ourselves or to others to get there, but there are *choices*.

Some people choose to keep their bad feelings. Bad feelings can be like a comfortable shoe that we have worn so often we want to keep. To break in a new pair is just too much effort. Some people would be uneasy about being happy. They haven't tried it and they are not about to. Other people like the revenge and the power that staying angry, guilty, or depressed gets them. These are all choices.

Much of our reluctance to being different is a version of fear. Figure out what you are afraid of and you have half the problem licked. Here are some thoughts about fears that might help:[1]

> ● *Fear increases in intensity in direct proportion to the amount of time you take to confront it.*
> (Have you ever delayed reporting a symptom, facing a conflict?) How long have you been avoiding something?

[1]We wish to acknowledge the following articles for their helpful ideas in preparing this section on fears: "Strategic/Pragmatic Aspects of Pain Management," by Jon Amundson, *Alberta Psychology*, Vol. 17, No. 1, 1988, pp. 3–6; and "Negative Explanation, Restraint and Double Description: A Template for Family Therapy," by Michael White, *Family Process*, Vol. 25, No. 2, June 1986, pp. 169–180.

What will happen if you avoid it for another two weeks, two months, two years?

- *Fear will wear different masks, particularly if it feels it is losing.*
  Fear will wear the mask of anger (fear that you will not be heard or respected); guilt (fear that you cannot live up to your own or others' expectations, that you have done something that is not repairable or forgivable); or despair (fear that you are powerless). What are you using to mask your fear?

- *Fear is contagious.*
  Any chance that you have simply caught it from someone? It's not hard when everyone is treating you as if you are a glass vase that might break at anytime. Courage is also contagious. Are you watching for people from whom you can catch courage? A nineteen-year-old told us that he got his act together by watching and talking to an eleven- year-old leukemic boy who taught him how not to be afraid and how the most important thing was how you lived each day.

- *Fear will take up as much of your life as you will give it.*
  How much of your life are you allowing it to take? Has it taken over your sleep, your appetite, your confidence, your friends? What is your limit as to how much it can have?

- *Fear cannot survive without good friends to feed it.*
  Fear needs a life support system, and that is a system of negative beliefs. Pessimism is a luxury you can't afford. What thoughts are you using to feed your fears? Are you exaggerating anything? Are you jumping ahead to what is coming or looking back at what you regret? Fear is rarely experienced in the present. It is most often an anticipation or a memory.

● *Fear is crushed by laughter.*
Two emotions cannot occupy the same space at the same time. When was the last time you laughed? Are you prepared to do anything about the lack of laughter in your life? We recognize that some people have a general rule against enjoying themselves. Laughter is not a compulsory action. Please feel free to stay miserable. We will not be offended.

● *Fear is conquered by hope.*
You may have to live with a disease, but you do not have to live with fear. How is your hope reservoir? What fills it up? What are you going to do about it?

We have all overcome some kind of fear previously. If we hadn't, would we ride on a roller coaster or a ferris wheel? We certainly wouldn't ride an elevator, get in a plane, or drive on the freeway (even as a passenger). We would never be able to cut our own fingernails or trust the toaster. These may be small fears, but if you have conquered even a small fear, think of the larger fear as just a little one that got away from you.

No one is expecting you to be without fears. The issue is how to deal with them. Here's our recipe:

1. Recognize that you have a history. Who you are today is a result of a lot of years. It takes time to change the computer program.

2. Start today. Stick with today. Yesterday is gone and tomorrow isn't here yet.

3. Start with yourself.

4. Decide what you would like different. You can start small. Notice how fear is involved.

5. Use your imaginary notebook or television to see yourself doing whatever you need to do to conquer the fear. Notice what it is and start practicing. Be open to learning whatever you need to in order to conquer your fear.

6. If possible, have a cheering section: someone who will notice the difference and be glad for you.

 If you fear you will suffer, you already suffer from your fear.

Adapted from Michel Eyquen De Montaigne

Go Jump in a Lake

Dealing with Anger

Agnes was a forty-year-old woman readmitted to the hospital for intravenous antibiotics to control a bacteria that repetitively grew in her lungs. Her strained smile was one I had seen many times during our talks. In addition to this life-long condition, she had also suffered for two-and-a-half years with an undiagnosed condition that was extremely painful and had required several surgeries. She was now unable to work. I asked, "Don't you ever get angry that your whole world has been turned upside down?"

She started to cry, trying to smile through her tears. She began to talk about what it felt like to be a spectator of life, rather than a participant — how there was a limit to the length of time a person can feel okay about being on the sidelines, how she felt set apart, that she was tired and frustrated at always being gracious about not doing the things that she loved to do, such as her skiing. It just was not the same sitting inside the lodge! She acknowledged she was indeed angry, but felt that she really had no right to be angry. After all, she was so much more fortunate than so many people. She had people who loved her and she had doctors who really cared. Who was there to be angry at?

Bill had been complaining of pain in his back and of weariness for a number of months. He had a few tests and was told to lose a few pounds. Weeks later, the diagnosis of a terminal disease was bitter news when a second opinion confirmed that his chances were very slim because of the late diagnosis.

Donnie was caught throwing eggs at the neighbor's windows. In his small community everyone knew that his father was dying. Donnie had never cried, never said he was scared. He had, however, become the toughest, hardest-hitting player on the hockey team and had actually hurt two players in the previous weeks. He had started to give his teachers a bad time, too. It was several talks later when he was able to admit he was really mad at his dad and God (if there was one) for the things his dad and he would never do — like the motorcycle trip they had talked of since he was little. It had been the dream that was going to make up for the years of his dad working away from home. Now nothing would make up for it.

Jessie's mother was dying. The family had been quite open about it. At age ten he had been told the realities about the situation, as had been his seven-year-old sister. The parents had requested a family session just to ensure that the children had an opportunity to talk. They seemed to be the model family in terms of what to say and do when a parent is dying. They were involved in hiking and camping for the summer and making the most out of the time they had with their mother. There seemed to be no resentment, no tears, no typical anticipatory grief about the whole issue. This seemed remarkable. However, to the question, 'What does your family do with 'sad,' " the seven-year-old piped up quickly and said, "Oh, that's easy. My brother just kicks me and I kick the dog."

Who do you kick? We may all *want* to kick when something is not the way we want it. Some people live with the illusion that the world is supposed to be the way that they want it to be and that if it isn't, they have a *right* to kick. The roots of resentment are in the beliefs we hold.

See if you recognize any of these:

- The world owes me health.

- It's not fair that I am sick; I should somehow be immune.

- If you love me, you should do what I want you to.

- The doctor has to care.

- There has to be an answer to everything.

- People have to be rational and reasonable.

- If you loved me, you would know what I need.

- Only sissies cry, so I will yell.

- People in this family are strong.

- If you can't say something nice, don't say anything at all.

The more of these you believe, the more likely you are to feel angry. Most people feel some degree of anger. What varies is the way people express anger. Each of us has our own style.

Perhaps you are a basic *tantrum thrower.* Tantrum throwers are the most entertaining. People around you may, however, be inhibited by flying kidney basins and foul language. Being a tantrum thrower has its advantages, the most obvious of which is that, if you have enough energy to throw a tantrum, you have enough energy to get well. Admittedly, getting well is not as entertaining, but then you have to be willing to sacrifice something. People tend to do two things if you are a tantrum thrower. They expose themselves only briefly to your abuse or they simply ignore the noise. If they are skilled in guilt induction, they will chastise you.

Or are you a basic *pouter*? The pouter is the person who seems to be perpetually annoyed at something. To be a good pouter, you have to have mastered the ability to keep frown lines on your forehead constantly. That way people are never sure why you are annoyed, but it keeps them cautious around you. The basic pouter doesn't have as much fun as the tantrum thrower. If you are a pouter, you were probably sent to your room when you had tantrums as a kid.

Maybe you fit into the category of the *"icer"*. The "icer" is master of the basic deep freeze techniques — you know, not saying anything. You don't have to. Other people can *feel* your anger. It is chilling. 'Icers" answer in controlled tones and clipped sentences and are undaunted by any humor. (If you're an "icer," you are likely to be reading Ivan Illich for bedtime entertainment.) People around you probably have a sense of being tolerated, but only just.

It is a shame to have a good "mad" interrupted. A good mad is healthy and definitely should be enjoyed. Instead, people usually start tiptoeing around. Just because you are angry, you may get treated as if you are fragile or as if you have just come down with the plague. The people around you probably don't understand that anger is a strong form of asking for something. Maybe you don't either.

Young Max was a university student headed for an exciting academic and professional career. That was Tuesday. On Wednesday he played football and became a quadriplegic. After months of "keeping his chin up," he was feeling the pressure of being able to do virtually nothing for himself. He found it very frustrating to have almost no privacy. He began to get cranky. His mother aggravated the situation by smothering him. He just wanted to be left alone more often. Couldn't she understand? Thankfully, after he admitted the difficulty, she could and did respect his need. If she hadn't, he, like many people, would have had not only his anger to deal with but also the guilt of knowing people were being cautious around him.

Not everyone is like Max's mother. Some people are threatened by anger and get defensive, as if the anger is an attack on them rather than a plea for something from the person who is angry. The situation deteriorates into an argument about who is right, rather than trying to understand what the anger means. Anger is too often used as a way for one person to win. Shouting matches take a lot of energy — something you don't have as much of when you are ill. Whoever wins the shouting match is thought to win the game, but if you watch closely, it is often the person who can walk away who has the power. You can't argue with someone who just isn't there!

Some people give in to an angry person. They say, "Okay, okay, I will do it," and then they don't. That's not any better as a solution. It just postpones the problem. So what *does* help?

First, check to see if anger is really what you are feeling. Sometimes we use anger to communicate a feeling that we are not good at communicating. It's as if anger is a mask for our real feelings. It's not uncommon to act angry when we are afraid or sad. Being scared doesn't feel so great if you pride yourself on being "tough." Tough people quite often express anger when they are scared. Many people find they end up crying when they are angry. The tears speak of the sadness or disappointment behind the anger.

Second, recognize that we all get angry at things sometimes. Anger is just one more way of us getting what we need. Anger might not always be the best way, but it sure beats depression. It is perfectly acceptable to say, "Look, I'm angry. I intend to be angry for a while. Don't bug me." There is no need to give all the reasons. Maybe it is even important that you *don't* itemize the reasons, because anger is not always rational and you don't want someone convincing you that you "shouldn't" be angry.

Anger can actually be fun! Having a friend who isn't scared or upset at your anger helps. One morning the secretary in my office was annoyed that the garbage had tipped over onto the floor. Aggravated, she began kicking the litter back into the container. It looked so satisfying that I joined her. Neither of us said a word. A few minutes later we both burst out laughing.

We need outlets for our anger. Anger is a natural response to situations where we are faced with more and more limitations and fewer and fewer options. When we get the anger out, there is more room for joy and caring. So get rid of the idea that anger is a NO-NO and get rid of the anger. The important issue is not whether you have anger but *where* you target it.

Anger is like a deep breath. You can't hold it forever. If you try, you will just feel as if you are going to explode, and then it will come out with an uncontrolled rush.

Jill was a soft-spoken florist who had difficulty accepting that she could even feel angry. She had worked for years for an unappreciative employer and said nothing. Only recently had she gained enough confidence to seek a position where she was paid more and treated more respectfully. She was preparing to move into her first home when she was told that she might die soon. She was so angry that she could hardly sleep at night. She needed an alternate outlet for her anger.

She returned to a session one day looking much lighter and wearing a smile. She had taken action with regard to her anger. She had gone into the part of town where there are a lot of secondhand shops and purchased boxes of cheap dishes. When she would become aware of her anger, she would SMASH as many as pleased her. Her mother, a delightful woman unafraid of emotional outbursts, would cheer and both would join in the clean up. Dishes are not the only option. Here are a few ideas that patients have shared with us over the years:

- Hang an old duffel bag stuffed with old linens or clothes where you will go by it often. Put a tennis racket beside it and enjoy smashing the duffel bag when you go by.

- Hang up a sign when you want to be alone.

- When having a "mad," hang up a sign up that says, "If you are intending on cheering me up, go home."

- Keep a piece of rubber hose beside your bed. Enjoy pounding.

- Write letters to people you are angry with and never send them.

- Think of how the situation would look in a cartoon.

- Send a "Thank you" note to the person you are mad at and stand by to watch how confused they become.

- Read a lot of cartoons.

- Spend money (preferably only if you have it).

- Get a massage.

- If you are well enough, play an aggressive sport.

- Beat the blazes out of the boss at golf.

- Stir-fry Chinese food so you get to cut up lots of things.

- Knead bread.

- Become an advocate for a downtrodden group so that you can write letter after letter to your senator or representative or member of the legislature.

- Have a "getting even" price list. What is any given frustration worth? One hour of tolerating George may be worth an uninterrupted bubble bath.

- Reward yourself for keeping your cool.

- Imagine telling someone what you really think of them.

- Every morning put a flower on the desk of someone you detest.

- Learn the relaxation response.

- Go to the mirror and say all the things you fantasize saying to whomever you are angry with.

- Cry.

- Paint with your kids' fingerpaints.

|| ● Talk it out with someone who will listen and care.

One part of anger is to recognize and express it. The second part is to do so *without causing injury to relationships*. You have to plan on the possibility that you will survive your illness, and you may want or need some people in your world when you are well. Here is a little formula that helps when expressing anger:

|| 1. Describe the situation.

|| 2. Describe your feelings.

|| 3. Describe what you want done or will be doing.

Here are some examples of what we mean. Follow along and then try a few of your own.

● "You come in every morning at 6:00 a.m. to take my temperature. My condition has nothing to do with a fever."
[*That's the situation; now for the feeling.*]
"I get frustrated because I am unable to go back to sleep."
[*Then what do you want done differently?*]
"I want to be allowed to sleep until I awake naturally."
[*If nothing changes, get more explicit.*]
"I will be asking the doctor to write an order NOT to wake me for a 6:00 a.m. temp," or, "I will refuse to have my temperature taken unless I am already awake. I will be cooperating with you at 7:30 when I normally awake."
[*Still no changes? It is time for more stringent measures.*]
"I will be asking to see the hospital administrator."

● "You promised to cut the lawn two days ago. You are well aware that I am unable to do so. I am feeling frustrated that it is still uncut, and I am feeling powerless to change that except to keep asking. I find it discouraging to be asking over and over. I would like to know

> if I can expect you to cut the lawn, and if your answer
> is "yes," I would like us to agree on when it will be cut.
> I am sure this is bugging you, too."

Practice makes perfect; one more for good measure.

> ● "You say I should take whatever time I need to recover,
> and yet you ask me daily when I will be back at work.
> I am feeling a little annoyed at not knowing what you
> really expect or what you really need from me. I would
> appreciate knowing what the situation with regard to
> my sick leave really is. That way we can minimize bad
> feelings."

Remember, anger can be healthy. It is part of our signal system. It is a way of telling us that something is not the way we want it. During an illness your basic rights, as well as your rights as a patient, can be violated. If it takes a little anger on your part to keep feeling like a valued human being, it is worth the energy. It is occasionally the only language that gets results. When you want something different, you have the responsibility of assessing whether that something is within your reach, and if so, by what means you want to get it. We hope anger is not your only choice, but it sure is a vital choice at times.

Institutions don't like anger. It is much noisier than sadness or depression or apathy. Angry people often say what they think, feel, and want. That's not always welcome. Don't forget that lots of professional caregivers don't like anger because not only does it mean more work for them, but it can also point out to them that they are not admitting the anger *they* have. How many bedpans can you empty in a day before you get frustrated? How many times can you have a patient die without feeling hurt or angry? Caregivers have to deny a lot of their feelings or they couldn't do their work. Caregivers are never intentionally insensitive. They will often regain their perspective if you ask, "If I was a member of your family, would you want me to be treated like this?" If you are sad, mad, or bad, it is just a bit more difficult for your caregivers to keep their professional masks on.

Trudi was middle-aged woman who was described as depressed. I saw her a couple of times, and she was very open about the reasons for her depression. Within a couple of days she started to assert herself with family and staff. A nurse stopped me in the hallway to inform me that our sessions had not worked, that now the patient was angry and asking for things. I assured the nurse that if, in a couple of days the patient was still "difficult," I would attempt to get her depressed again.

I understood most of your message, but would you mind repeating that last scream?

Ashleigh Brilliant

© Ashleigh Brilliant
Santa Barbara, California

You Have the Right to Remain Silent

Dealing with Depression

When I go to a cocktail party, someone skilled in the social graces always has to ask, "And what do you do?" They always seem to be the same people who know how to balance a glass of punch, a piece of cheese, a large strawberry, and a clump of grapes all in one hand! When I used to reply, "I work for the government," that occasionally satisfied them. But more often than not, I was pushed to answer the sequel, "What do you do for government?" When I replied, "I am a psychologist," a good number graciously excused themselves to get another drink! Some pushed on without the good grace to recognize my reluctance, until I said, "I work with the seriously ill, a high percentage of whom die." The classic response was, "Oh, that must be depressing." Sometimes I had the energy to give a long harangue about why it was not depressing, and sometimes I simply commented, "It is not without its challenges." More often they seem satisfied with the latter.

One physician I know decided she wanted to avoid being asked questions about her work while on a fishing trip. When she was asked about her career, she reported loudly that she was a mortician. It worked so well that the next summer, at the same lodge, she repeated the procedure. The new proprietor was delighted and added, "Perhaps you would like to meet the gentlemen at the next table. All four of them are morticians, too." Puzzled, she turned her head, only to recognize them as dentists with whom she had fished the previous summer!

What do visitors and family ask on the sly? "How are his spirits?" "Is she depressed?" What they may really be saying is that they would likely be depressed under similar circumstances. They don't know what to say or how to help. Of course, they don't ask either.

Depression is the most overused, misunderstood word in our psychological jargon.

One morning I was accompanying the entourage of professionals and budding professionals on "rounds." That's the morning ritual where anywhere from four to eight persons, only one of whom you vaguely know as your admitting physician, come into your room at 7:00 a.m. while the sleeping medication you didn't want hasn't worn off yet. There are brief introductions that don't match names to faces. Your permission to be invaded is not solicited. It seems you are to view this violation of normal courtesy as a privileged opportunity to contribute to medical education.

This particular morning, the informal lesson was about depression. The physician turned to the eager interns accompanying him and said, "Now the woman we are going to see next is depressed." My ears perked up! The learning process continued. "The way that you know someone is depressed is that you get bored talking to them." End of lesson! I stopped going to rounds! (Now you know part of the reason why I keep saying some physicians seem ill-equipped to handle the emotional side of illness.)

What is this thing called depression? It is first important to know what depression is NOT. Depression is not sadness. Sadness is a natural response to the experience of loss. When you are sad, there is a sense of missing what you have lost, whether it is a pet, a job, a body function, or a dream. There is a sense of reluctantly having to say, "Goodbye." Sadness is a feeling that leads to healing. It is natural — we see it even in the animal world.

Depression is not just tiredness. When people are sick with the flu, no one expects them to entertain visitors or make important decisions. We accept that they are not feeling well and that they need their rest. As a matter of fact, if they go out when they are exhausted, we berate them for not looking after themselves. We don't worry about someone with a short-term illness getting depressed. But when the illness is chronic, the rules and expectations seem to change.

It is natural to have down days. That is not depression. Depression is nature's way of giving us a break from feeling. It is a state of not caring about things. If you are sad, hurting, discouraged, resentful, you are at least feeling. When you are depressed, there is a sense of "not feeling."

Depression is a collection of symptoms that, if they persist long enough, is labeled "depression." There are both physical and psychological signs for which to watch.

One common sign of depression is a change in eating habits, usually in the form of loss of appetite. However, when you are ill, many things can affect appetite. It's not surprising that your appetite changes when you are on thirty doses of this and that: This helps you sleep, that helps you wake up; this helps your appetite, that helps your bowels; this helps your inflammation, that helps your pain. It is no wonder you are full by lunch. Therefore, loss of appetite does not necessarily signal depression, but it is one sign to watch for.

If you are prone to overweightness, with your luck, your change in eating habits could be toward the less common direction of an increased appetite. One woman reported being so depressed after realizing what her diagnosis really meant, she sat down and ate four gigantic bowls of ice cream. She didn't realize what she was doing until she was scraping the bottom of the last bowl. What was amazing was that she didn't even *like* ice cream!

Difficulty sleeping, or sleeping much more than usual (as if to avoid something), are also clues to depression. So are reduced energy, slowness of speech, and lack of motivation. The problem is that these same things are also signs of illness. If you are healthy and complain of these signs, they are much more likely to be symptomatic of depression than if you are struggling with a life-threatening and exhausting illness. In other words, the signs of depression are hard to distinguish from the signs of sickness.

If you are honest with yourself, you will probably know if you are depressed. Are you crying more? Losing your temper more often? Not able to concentrate? Indecisive? Have no interest in anything? Nothing seems to give you pleasure? It might be depression; then again, it might not be. Remember, these things may be caused by illness and medications, too. Tell your doctor about them and ask if the difference in your feelings could be due to the illness or to the side-effects of drugs you are taking. There are numerous conditions and medications that can send you into the doldrums. (See the chapter "Hold On — Help Is on the Way," page 157, for a discussion of depression that occurs on a biochemical basis.)

The depression that you personally can do something about has its roots in how you are thinking. Are you starting to question if people care? Are you feeling worthless and a burden to others? Feeling inadequate? (Or at least more inadequate than usual?) Feeling guilty about things you are doing, or not doing, or that you did years ago? Even entertaining the idea that the world might be a better place without you?

Thinking about suicide is not as uncommon as you might think. You are not the first one to think about how you could ease the burden of those who care, perhaps even ease the financial cost. You may even feel that, if you have to live this way, life has no meaning and you might as well be dead. The trouble with suicide is that it is something you cannot redecide tomorrow. Thinking about it is not necessarily wrong or unhealthy. Planning for it and acting on it is likely a sign of depression. There are exceptions, though.

Ted was a hard-driving, straight-from-the-shoulder oil worker, who had a tale to tell about every place in the world he had worked. Whatever else Ted had, he had character, and he took pride in being a "man." Home care staff was worried about whether Ted had a boa constrictor in his room and a gun in his bedside table. While he was in the hospital with neither, it seemed the ideal time to talk to him. I decided to be as direct as he seemed to be, so I said, "Ted, some of us are worried about what having a gun in your bedside table might mean? Have you had any thoughts about doing yourself in?"

Ted retorted, "Who wouldn't? That's why I keep it there, and if you take it away, I *will* find a way to do myself in. As long as that gun is there, I know I am a man. I know I have the courage to face this damn disease. You take that gun away and you've told me I am a coward, that you don't think I am man enough to handle this."

I suggested to home care that if the boa constrictor gave them any problem, they should shoot it with the revolver. Ted died of his disease, endeared to us all.

People will take a variety of approaches to get you out of a depression. The "Coach Approach" folks are the "And-how-are-we-today?" people. The message is, "Let's be up all the time, no matter how lousy the situation is." They interfere with the natural process of grieving a loss.

Harvey had recently received the news that, not only was he dying, but that he would be paralyzed from the waist down until the end of his days. In other words, he was adjusting to some very challenging changes in his life! When I came in, he said, 'If you intend to say what a nice day it is, and ask how my breakfast was, you can leave. I don't care how nice it is. I can't go out in it, and I have always hated breakfast." I promised to be appropriately somber, and we laughed for an hour as he described how everyone was bent on him rallying. They would pull up his blinds, say cheerful things, but never say, 'Harve, how is it for you?'" As far as he was concerned, they were trying to coach him in a game where they were not even on the field.

Then there are the "You've-got-to-do-it-for-US" folks. Some of them are so good at this that they should get the Guiness Book of Records Award for Guilt Induction. We have seen patients hang on for weeks in unbelievable agony, so that their loved ones wouldn't feel as if they were failures in instilling the will to live. What some people fail to realize is that, for the patient, there is a point when dying does not feel like the worst thing that can happen.

It can get depressing to feel as if, even during the last days of your life, people will not let you be you. They insist that you keep on pretending. You may begin to wish it was all over so you could take off your mask of courage. When you are depressed, you don't feel like being patronized, cajoled, or humored.

Still other people approach depression by getting scared and going away. That may be a welcome peace for a while, but it can get very lonely when you are depressed. If you are aware that you are somewhat depressed, try to let people know that you are struggling and that you do want them to care, even if you are not able to respond at this time. We recover from most bouts of depression. In the interim you could put up a small sign above your bed:

Stand by. I will be back as soon as I can figure out how to get out of this black hole.

Sometimes we need to shut down because we're just not ready to deal with our feelings. If you are angry, you may need to stop feeling altogether for a while until you find a way to ventilate your anger. In other circumstances, you may feel so discouraged that if you felt the full force of the discouragement, it would be too much, so you just shut down the whole feeling system for a while.

If symptoms of depression persist, it is time to ask for help. You wouldn't walk around with a broken leg for long, would you? Why go around with a broken psyche? Effective help is available. Depression is not something you need to hide or be ashamed of: It is not uncommon for a person who has had a series of physical and emotional challenges to experience depression. There can be just too much happening in too short a time. However, you do need to watch for signs of being shut down too long. There is no right or wrong amount of time, but we recommend that you not stay down too long.

You may also be able to avoid some depression. Do your best to think constructively. If possible, stay physically active. (You can pass on the racquetball.) Keep some routine in your life. Unless you are confined to bed, get dressed every day, continue to take pride in your personal grooming. Maintain some social contact, but avoid anyone who gets you down. Avoid getting overtired. Who doesn't feel down when they're tired?

Break big problems down into little problems, and then attack the little ones. Feeling overwhelmed is one of the most effective ways of getting and staying depressed. Have short term goals. Make your goals things that are within your control and be sure to reward yourself for achieving them. You don't help yourself if you make a list of ten things, get nine of them done, and then berate yourself for the one that is left! Make simple, accomplishable goals.

Something to look forward to helps, too. It can be a holiday, a visit somewhere, new clothes, whatever. Plan something in your life that you can anticipate with pleasure. No matter how you are feeling there is something that, if it happened, would help you feel better.

One widower, who was experiencing not only the loss of his wife but also the loss of many of his lifetime friends, reported, "Everyday I start out by checking the obituaries. If I'm not listed, I have at least one thing to be thankful for during the day!"

Laughter helps. Spending sprees help, if you have money. (If you don't, you'll be more depressed later.) Helping someone else helps. How about buying an ice cream for that little kid who comes for treatment the same time you do?

If you are concerned that you might be prone to depression, talk with someone you trust. Choose the person(s) carefully. You need an ear, not a mouth. Tell them how you are feeling and what your life is like for you right now. Assure them you do not expect them to make it different. You just want to share it with someone.

If people keep patronizing you with, "Oh, you'll be fine," but on the inside you know you are not fine, get to someone who is knowledgeable and helpful. If your feelings of depression persist despite your efforts, seek out a professional. There are times when self-help or the support of a friend are not enough. Sometimes talking to someone outside of the situation helps. The professional is not caught up in the personalities and can offer unbiased viewpoints. If you feel you would benefit from help in this area, ask for a referral. You may want to check out their credentials, too.

Keep in mind that not all professionals are trained to help with the emotional aspects of illness. If you get an advice-giving, opinion-ated helper, fire them. Get one who listens. A professional will help sort out whether there is a physical or chemical reason for your depres-sion. Remember, it may not be "in your head" at all.

Pat yourself on the back for recognizing what would be helpful. Let go of the nonsense that you have to do it all alone.

Don't worry if you *don't* get depressed. It's not a requirement. Elsie had had a mastectomy almost a year before she came to counsel-ing. She wanted cancer out of her life. She was back working and running her home, her marriage was good, but she just wished that she would get depressed. Yes, you read it correctly. You see, her doctor had said, "You'll get depressed before this is all over." Who knows what the doctor really meant, but Elsie had taken him literally. She thought it could not be all over until she had been depressed, so she hoped that the darn depression would get there soon so that she could have the depression, get over it, and have illness out of her life.

What do you do if someone caring for you gets depressed? Give them this chapter. Why not the whole book?

If you are a person who's usually depressed and like what it gets you, we don't want to interfere with your lifestyle. Please don't feel that you have to give it up. Just tell those you care about some of the ideas in this chapter because, if you are depressed all the time, they will need them!

 What makes things so difficult is that I have never been at this point in life before.

Ashleigh Brilliant

Pardon Me
and I'll Pardon You

Dealing with Guilt

Many seriously ill patients feel responsible for their illness and are constantly apologizing for having to impose on others for their care. Sound familiar? It's not your fault that you are ill! You didn't wake up one morning and say to yourself, "I think I'd like to have a fatal disease today!" So why do you feel that you have to apologize? If your caretakers were the ones who were the patients, would you do any less for them than they do for you? Of course not!

It's natural to feel a little guilty about things you may have thought or said about someone who is now extending considerable kindness to you, thereby proving you wrong. You're probably not the only one feeling guilty. They may feel guilty that they can't do enough, that you are sick rather than they, or perhaps, as children often think, that they have contributed to your illness.

Children are particularly prone to magical thinking. A child may be angry about being disciplined and say,"I hate you! I wish you were dead!" Then when the person really does become ill, they think that they are responsible.

Those caring for you may even think that they deserve to be the sick one because of something they have done in the past for which they have not yet been able to forgive themselves. They may not even be aware of their guilt.

Clara was a fifty-two-year-old woman who came to the office because of severe Raynaud's Disease. This is a disease in which the arteries in the fingers and hands go into spasm with minimal exposure to cold. Various treatments had been tried with no effect. The tips of her fingers all had scars on them because of the death of some of the tissue after repeated episodes of arterial spasm and the associated loss of blood supply.

She was in constant pain and wished to learn hypnosis to control some of the pain, and possibly the spasm as well. She proved to be a good hypnotic subject and was able to control a good deal of her pain. She was not aware of any past event that might have contributed in any way to her present illness. Just to be sure, hypnotic age regression was tried to see if there might be any events in her past which might be contributing factors.

Under hypnosis, she remembered an episode which happened at age five. In her town it had been the custom for neighborhoods to have block dances. The entire city block would be barricaded off, a band hired, and a keg of beer acquired. All the neighbors would chip in, and a good time would be had by all. At one of these block parties, Clara's parents had been unable to get a baby sitter and, since the party was just in front of their house, had told Clara to baby-sit for her younger sister who was still in diapers. The parents said they would pop into the house every so often to make sure that everything was all right.

Shortly after one of the occasions when her parents had looked in, Clara's sister filled her diaper. She did such a good job that it spilled out onto the floor as she walked about. Clara knew that she should clean up after her sister and took a cloth and tried to mop up the mess. Being only five, she was not very good at cleaning and only succeeded in smearing the mess around.

Just then her father returned and found her on her knees smearing stool around the floor. He immediately assumed that she was making a deliberate mess and proceeded to squeeze each of her hands very hard and then slap them saying, "Bad girl! Bad girl!"

Clara naturally felt very bad and, briefly hating him for unjustly punishing her, wished him dead. Shortly thereafter her father was killed in an industrial accident, and Clara assumed it was her fault. Her unconscious mind had been punishing her for this unforgivable act ever since!

Eventually Clara was able to bring her adult understanding and insight to bear on this painful memory. She was then able to forgive herself for having briefly wished her father dead. She also knew that she had no part in his accidental death and could stop punishing herself.

Her hands improved and the pain relented but, naturally, the scars at the tips of her fingers remained.

This case was particularly interesting because Clara did not even know that she was punishing herself. What about you? Is there anything for which you should forgive yourself? Or is there anyone whom you should forgive for having done something to you? Holding on to anger or resentment is just as harmful as believing that you deserve to be continually punished. The person at whom you're angry doesn't feel a thing, but you end up with the heartburn and the headache. It simply is not worth it! Consider declaring a blanket amnesty for everyone who has ever offended you in any way. You'll feel much better for it!

While you're at it, forgive yourself and give yourself permission to get well again. "How do I do this?" you're asking? Simple! Close your eyes and imagine the little person inside you. Inside each of us is a little Susan, Fred, or Clara. Feel that little child's arms around your neck. Feel the child's warm breath on your cheek. Hear that little child say, "Thank you for remembering that I exist! Thank you for remembering my needs as well! I love you too!"

Take that little child on an imaginary walk in your favorite place. Tell that child the things he or she needs to hear. Let the child tell you the things you need to know as well. See that child smile at you. Then imagine that the child goes back inside of you. See the child going into the control room that controls the way you feel and the way your body works! See the child adjusting the switches and dials so that everything operates smoothly, so that you feel well! See yourself getting healthier and stronger.

Each time you practice relaxing, even for an instant, that child will know you're looking in on him or her, that you care. And that child will reciprocate by caring for you as well!

Once you've learned to forgive yourself, as well as others, you can direct all your attention to getting well again rather than to harboring old resentments. If you're having trouble forgiving yourself, talk to someone you can trust, such as a counselor, a member of the clergy, or a trustworthy relative or friend. It really helps!

Mabel was sixty-eight and had been married for forty-three years. She had had nightmares almost all of her married life, so much so, that all of the family knew about them, and she refused to visit anywhere lest she embarrass herself in someone else's home by screaming out during the night. The nightmares had begun following an affair she had had early in her marriage. She had never been able to tell anyone about the affair because of her shame. When she was finally able to tell a counselor about it, her nightmares stopped! If only she had been able to do that much earlier, she would have spared herself forty years of torment!

IF MABEL CAN FORGIVE HERSELF, SO CAN YOU!

A good way to begin forgiving yourself is to start by forgiving someone else for having done something to you. Many years ago I was punished for breaking a valuable vase when I was completely innocent. It's curious that I was not angry at whoever really did break the vase, but I did harbor a grudge for a long time about being punished unfairly. If it happened once, I thought, it could happen again. It was a real relief when I was able to forgive my parents for having punished me. At that point I no longer had to continually fear being punished unfairly again in the future.

How about you? Want to try forgiving somebody right now?

     Life is an adventure in forgiveness.

Norman Cousins

SECTION 6

BODY

Hold On — Help Is on the Way

Why Do I Feel So Crappy When I'm Constipated?

Coping with Side Effects

Whenever you are ill, a change occurs in the normal functioning of your body. In the case of an acute illness such as the flu, certain cells in your body produce chemicals designed to destroy the invading virus. Among these chemicals are interferon and interleukin, which are also being used to treat certain cancers. These chemicals cause fever, muscle aching, and the loss of appetite commonly associated with acute infectious illnesses. Small wonder that you feel crappy when you have the flu! However, what you're really feeling is your body fighting back against the invading agent.

In the case of chronic illness, many of these mechanisms work in the same way. Your body produces chemicals intended to fight off invaders, but often this response is ineffectual and only serves to weaken you further. In the case of advanced cancer, some of these chemicals can cause severe loss of appetite and weakness. There is an individual variability in how each person responds to these chemicals in their body, but anyone who receives an injection of these chemicals in a sufficient dosage will immediately lose their appetite and feel ill.

The same production of chemicals intended to protect the body, but actually causing it harm, applies to many other chronic illnesses, as well, including arthritis, diabetes, inflammatory bowel disease, and AIDS. In the case of AIDS, certain blood cells, in their attempt to combat the AIDS virus, actually produce chemicals harmful to the body as a whole.

Your body has been healing itself all of your life. Cell renewal is a natural process. Similarly, in the case of cancer chemotherapy or radiotherapy, your body is programmed to repair itself and allow you to feel better. If all goes according to plan, and given enough time, your body will completely recover from the side effects of chemotherapy or radiotherapy.

In order to understand some of the side effects of both cancer and its treatment, it is necessary to understand certain basic principles. *Principle number one is that cancer cells grow more slowly than normal white cells and many tissue cells.* That's right, more slowly. The average doubling time for a cancer cell can vary between 70 and 260 hours, whereas the doubling time for normal white cells is 18 hours (39 hours, for normal cells of the gastrointestinal tract).

Principle number two is that chemotherapy and radiotherapy injure both normal and cancer cells, causing certain percentages of them to be damaged and killed. But because healthy cells recover long before cancer cells do, after an interval of time, the normal cells proceed to replenish themselves before the cancer cells have a chance to do so. It is rather like walking down a staircase: The normal cells bounce back to the top of the staircase after each treatment cycle, while the cancer cells continue to be damaged progressively by each additional treatment. The cancer cells eventually end up at the bottom of the stairs, while the healthy cells are at the top.

This means that repeated courses of therapy can be given at intervals long enough to permit normal tissue cells to recover and short enough to prevent the cancer cells from doing the same.

After each course of chemotherapy or radiotherapy, your doctor will check your white cell count or platelet count to see whether your healthy cells have bounced back to the top of the stairs and whether you can safely receive another cycle of treatment which will cause further and progressive damage to any remaining cancer cells.

Unfortunately, at the present time we don't have any chemotherapy agents that are smart enough to target only cancer cells for attack. That's why your mouth transiently becomes sore or why you may develop diarrhea for a few days after getting chemotherapy. The healthy cells have to suffer temporarily.

But help is on the way! There are already certain immuno-therapy agents that have the ability to attack only tumor cells. Research is also underway to link specific antibodies to chemotherapy agents. These antibodies seek out and attach themselves only to cancer cells, thus allowing the chemotherapy agents to kill only cancer cells. If this approach is validated by current research, furture chemotherapy will be much more specific and less associated with side effects.

So far we have talked about feeling crappy with cancer, but you can feel just as rotten with any chronic disease, such as arthritis, diabetes, or AIDS. Despite all of the physical reactions, your attitude has a great deal to do with how you feel and act, even though you may be seriously ill.

We've discussed the importance of attitude in relation to chronic disease in the chapter "The Altitude of Your Attitude" (page 52). (You may want to go back and take a look at this chapter again.) In a similar fashion, any negative emotion such as guilt, fear, or depression will reduce your body's ability to defend itself.

Monitor your stress level. There is good evidence to show that stress has a deleterious effect on the immune system and the body as a whole. Excessive stress produces increased production of adrenal hormones, such as cortisone and adrenalin. These can interfere with normal immune function, both in terms of the amounts of circulating immune cells and their functioning. This particularly important for people who have AIDS.

And, above all, remember how important it is to give yourself a reason to live, not to die. What about all your loved ones? They're counting on you. "What loved ones?" did you ask? Why, all the loved ones you haven't even met yet!

Stick around; there's a lot more coming than you can even imagine! There are people waiting even now to discover you! Just as you've discovered us! (Besides, you haven't even written us a note to tell us what you think of this book yet!)

"Do I have to do all this myself?" you ask. Nope! Turn to the next chapter. We'll help!

The only requirement for getting there is to keep on going.

Alexander Levitan

Hold On —
Help Is on the Way!

Pain and Symptom Management

Guess what's the most important thing about getting help when something is bothering you! YOU HAVE TO ASK FOR IT !!!

They stopped teaching mind-reading in medical school several years ago. If something is bothering you, talk to someone about it! This includes physical as well as psychological issues. If you can't bring yourself to discuss it outright, write a note. But for goodness sake, TELL SOMEONE!

Some people feel that to admit that they're having pain is a sign of weakness or defeat. Nonsense! Pain is a very valuable signal that tells you that something needs attention. However, once the pain signal has alerted you to the problem, the pain loses its utility. At that point it's perfectly reasonable to take whatever measures are necessary to eliminate, or at least modify, the pain. Ignoring or tolerating pain makes no sense.

The story is told about the Marine drill sergeant who was exhorting his trainees about the true meaning of becoming a Marine. "Marines are men! Marines don't know the meaning of the word pain!" he told his men with great emphasis. To illustrate his point, he looked around in the grass surrounding the training area and found a large snapping turtle slowly lumbering its way along.

He picked up the snapping turtle and, prying its jaws open, allowed it to attach itself to his nose. With the turtle hanging there, he turned to his platoon and said, "See what a Marine can do! Marines don't know the meaning of the word pain!"

At that point he picked up an old bottle lying nearby and struck the snapping turtle sharply on the head. The startled turtle let go its grip and fell to the ground, eventually crawling off in the grass. The drill sergeant turned to the assembled troops and asked, "Any of you want to try that?"

There was a pause, then one recruit way in the back timidly raised his hand and said, "Aaallright, but don't hit me too hard with the bottle!"

You're not a Marine, and you don't have anything to prove to anyone. If you're having pain or if you're not feeling well, ask for help! There is no such thing as a hypochondriac with a serious illness! If you don't tell your doctor what's going on, your doctor can't help you and will probably assume that all is going well.

Let's talk about a few specifics. Three of the problems most commonly encountered by seriously ill patients are pain, nausea, and depression.

PAIN

Pain is one of the primary concerns of many seriously ill patients. It doesn't have to be! Just about every medical facility has a pain clinic or a group of individuals especially trained to deal with acute and chronic pain. Even the most advanced and intense pain can be controlled with an appropriate dose of continuous infusion morphine which can readily be arranged for you, even in your home.

There is also currently available a series of venous access devices, things that allow doctors to be able to draw blood and give intravenous medications without even having to stick a needle into you. These look like tiny soft plastic tubes and are inserted under local anesthesia very easily. Generally this is one of the first things that is done before starting therapy if frequent drawing of blood samples will be required or if you will need frequent infusions of intravenous fluids or medications.

These devices are simple to maintain and generally require only periodic flushing with a saline solution to keep them from being blocked by blood clots. They are readily removable when they are no longer needed.

In addition, they are all easily connected to a series of portable pumps which are about the size of a pack of cards and can be worn attached to your belt or clothing. The pumps can be set so that they can operate for up to a week without being refilled or having the batteries changed. (Sorry, they don't come in fashion-coordinated colors!)

As long as we're discussing fancy electrical devices, you may already know about T.E.N.S. units. (T.E.N.S. stands for Transcutaneous Electrical Nerve Stimulating units; but you knew that, didn't you!) They send a tiny electrical current through electrodes attached to your skin. This current is barely noticeable, but it blocks your brain's ability to recognize pain signals, and any pain present is substantially reduced. Pretty slick, huh?

The electrodes look like tiny band-aids and have adhesive on the side which attaches to your skin. (In case you are afraid that there is a needle hiding somewhere, there isn't.) The T.E.N.S. units work particularly well in relieving post-operative pain and pain of musculoskeletal origin, such as whiplash, pinched nerves, and severe sprains.

A simplified version of T.E.N.S. that does not use batteries at all is becoming available. This model uses galvanic current developed by placing two dissimilar metals next to each other, and it costs almost nothing.

Other techniques are available, including permanent and temporary nerve blocks which can be performed by most recently-trained anesthesiologists. Similarly, new formulations of time-release preparations of morphine are readily available, as well as rectal morphine suppositories for persons who cannot take medications orally. (The only trick is to remember to remove the tin-foil before inserting them!)

Maybe you've heard the story about the lady who was instructed by her doctor to collect a twenty-four hour urine sample. She called her doctor at 2:00 a.m. and said, "Doctor, it's been twenty-two hours, and I don't think I can stand it any longer!"

NAUSEA

After that story, it's time to talk about nausea. Nausea can be caused by a variety of things, including excessive stomach acid, direct or indirect effect of drugs, or emotions. With regard to the latter, many patients are troubled by "anticipatory emesis." This means that they become nauseated when they even begin to *think* about coming to the doctor's office or the chemotherapy clinic.

You've heard of Pavlov, a Russian physician, and how he trained dogs to salivate at the sound of a bell because they associated this sound with being fed? Well, anticipatory emesis is the same thing. Patients associate a visit to the doctor with the receipt of drugs which have nauseated them in the past and, as a consequence, develop nausea even before arriving in the doctor's office.

If you don't believe in this, ask the doctor who, a year after treatment had ended, greeted a former patient in the theater row in which the doctor was about to take a seat. The patient vomited as he stood up to let the doctor into the row.

Behavior modification, which involves learning new techniques to alter your behavior, and hypnosis are both very effective in dealing with nausea, as well as with pain. We'll be discussing self-hypnosis in a later chapter, but feel free to peek ahead if you like.

A story illustrative of how *not* to deal with the problem of nausea goes like this:

> A patient called her oncologist and said, "You know, Doc, every time I come to your office, I become nauseated even before I get my chemotherapy! I feel fine in the car, but just as soon as I get into your office, I begin to feel sick!"
>
> "No problem," said the doctor, "I'll just ask my nurse to come down and give you your chemotherapy in your car. Just call and tell us when you're leaving home, and the nurse will meet you in the parking lot."
>
> It was arranged for the patient to receive the chemotherapy in this fashion, and everything seemed to be going well until the patient called and said, "You know, Doc, every time I get into my car I feel nauseated!"

The best way to prevent anticipatory nausea is to see to it that you never experience nausea in the first place. If you have never had nausea in association with chemotherapy, you cannot anticipate what has never been experienced! The way to achieve this is to use a combination of effective antinauseants currently available. These generally include metaclopramide (Reglan) given at frequent intervals after chemotherapy, usually in combination with dexamethasone (Decadron) and lorazepam (Ativan). The latter agent even makes you forget the whole experience. Sorry to tell you, smoking pot is passé. We now have the active ingredient tetra-hydro-cannabinol in capsule form, but other agents are even more effective. Don't get depressed about giving up pot smoking. We are going to talk about depression right now.

DEPRESSION

You have probably already read the chapter on the subject of depression ("You Have the Right to Remain Silent," page 141), but let's talk a little more about it now.

In the setting of chronic illness, depression can occur purely on a biochemical basis. Chronic illness is a constant stress on your body and results in the overproduction of stress-related hormones, such as adrenalin and cortisone. This often results in the depletion of the chemical building blocks used to make these hormones (and, incidentally, many other hormones, including those necessary for the brain to function normally). It is this deficiency of certain chemicals in the brain, such as nor-epinephrine and serotonin, that results in depression. Without these chemicals, messages are not transmitted properly from one part of the brain to another.

Depressing, isn't it? No, it isn't, because treatment is readily available if you tell your doctor about the symptoms and ask for help. The usual symptoms of depression include weepiness, excessive fatigue, early morning awakening, insomnia, constipation, and a lack of interest in anything.

The treatment can be chemical, psychological, or both. Chemical treatment of depression consists of drugs which restore the brain's supply of the deficient chemicals These are called antidepressants and, taken daily, will begin to work within several days and reach maximum effect within four to six weeks. Like vitamin pills given to a vitamin-deficient patient, don't expect them to work immediately. Similarly, once they are discontinued, their benefit will persist for several weeks.

Thus, if you're feeling depressed, remind yourself that you didn't cause it to happen. Like a vitamin deficiency, your body is missing something it needs to function normally, and you need to correct the deficiency in order to feel good.

Just as antidepressants are appropriate under certain circumstances, so too psychotherapy can effectively help you deal with the stresses which can lead to depression and is often sufficient to correct the problem. In addition, new drugs and non-drug methods of treating pain, nausea, and depression are constantly being developed and modified. Your physician or therapist can best keep you updated in this regard.

The name of the game is to get to tomorrow.

Ronna Fay Jevne

Two Straws, Please

Staying Sensual and Sexual

Everyone's rules about sex differ. The topic is a personal and a sensitive one. But sex is a natural expression of our needs to love and to be loved, so let's talk about it.

It's hard to be sexy when you're in pain or nauseated or feeling extremely fatigued. But, thank goodness, those physical deterrents occur only rarely. That leaves you all the rest of the time to be sexy.

There's no reason why you can't have just as satisfying a sex life now as you had before you became ill. You may not make love as often, but the feelings of intimacy can be just as good, if not better! And it can mean a whole lot more. It did for Max and Sally.

Sally and Max had been married for thirty-six years and had gotten into the habit of making love almost every night as a way of saying good-night to each other. Then Sally developed severe diabetes which eventually resulted in the amputation of one of her legs.

Sally became severely depressed and experienced intense pain in her stump almost each night after Max went home at the end of visiting hours. Sally finally admitted that she was very apprehensive about whether Max would continue to love her now that her leg was gone. She was afraid that Max wouldn't be interested in making love to a one-legged lady.

With Sally's permission, her concerns were brought to Max's attention. Max pointed out that when he went home at night, he didn't take his love with him but rather left it with her to keep forever, just as he would always have her love with him. That reassurance took care of the stump pain which no longer occurred as soon as visiting hours were over.

But the depression remained until the therapist gave them

permission to think about new and more creative ways to make love under their new circumstances. Max came in one day with some diagrams tucked under his arm. He waited for a moment alone with Sally and then showed her his drawings. He had figured out a whole series of new and different ways they could make love, now that they didn't have Sally's other leg to worry about! Sally could hardly wait to get home. . .and did so soon.

It's interesting how one's self-image profoundly affects one's sexuality. Perhaps you know of someone who might not be considered beautiful but who is very sensual and alluring sexually. It's also nice to discover that, at social gatherings, the person you came with is still the most attractive one there — from your point of view.

Even if you don't have a Max at home, you can still enjoy moments of intimacy and tenderness. If you don't feel like making mad, passionate love, you can still enjoy a sensual massage, complete with flavored or scented massage oil, and can reciprocate by doing the same for your partner. Sometimes a foot rub feels as good as a belly rub!

Studies have shown that even animals need to be touched and cuddled in order to remain healthy. That's why baby gorillas and chimps in zoos are sent home in diapers with their caretakers. We all need to be touched and caressed in order to maintain continuity with our senses and our humanity. Studies with obstetric patients have shown that just touching the patient during labor can significantly reduce the patient's blood pressure, pulse, and discomfort during labor.

Sometimes partners are reluctant to bring up the subject of sex for fear that sex will unduly tire their loved one. So it will be up to you to be a little more forward than usual and to discuss more openly the needs of both you and your partner. Should you be too tired for sex, just giving your partner permission to masturbate with or without your help is often sufficient. If it seems appropriate, experiment with vibrators or rent an erotic film to help out!

Whether you need to improve or modify your sex life, be sure that you discuss it frankly and sincerely with your partner. If it's difficult to discuss the subject with your partner, talk to your doctor about it.

To introduce the subject with a little humor to see if your doctor will pick up on it, you might try this:

"Doc, my wife and I have had a lot of hard times, but we've always gotten through them and usually with no hard feelings. Well, now I've got some trouble with a different kind of 'no hard feelings.' Got any ideas?"

Well, if you're having trouble with "no hard feelings," talk to your doctor about it and help may be forthcoming.

If your doctor seems uncomfortable about discussing the matter, ask if you can be referred to someone who is trained to deal with human sexuality issues.

There are a variety of prosthetic devices that make sex satisfying and enjoyable when a man has been rendered impotent by his therapy. One technique involves a simple, self-administered injection that results in a normal and durable erection. There are also new surgical procedures that accomplish the same therapeutic goals by implanting silicone rubber rods or inflatable balloons that enable previously impotent men to have normal and satisfying erections.

It may even be that your doctor can help with some symptom that has made lovemaking difficult, such as impotence after a radical prostatectomy or dryness of the vagina after a total hysterectomy. Remember: What your doctor doesn't know about you, he or she can't help you with. The same applies to your partner.

Communication and understanding are also important to a satisfactory sexual relationship in order to understand and fulfill mutual expectations. If you would like your partner to try something different, be sure that you both understand what you have in mind.

And, by the way, there's nothing wrong with lying by the fire with your head in someone's lap while that person strokes your hair. Similarly, a good back rub or foot rub can feel very sensual without being sexual, unless you want it to be.

In addition, when you're seriously ill, you become more aware of all the beauty surrounding you, as you become more aware that it might not always be available to you. Enjoy the lovely colors of a sunset or the fragile beauty of a flower petal. Revel in the fragrance of a rose or the tender call of a loon for its mate. Become so involved in life that every moment is an eternity of sensation and pleasure.

Many patients have said that it's a shame that they had to develop a fatal disease in order to learn how to appreciate life. By being able to dispense with the trivial aspects of life, they are able to appreciate what is truly meaningful. It's as if all their senses are heightened.

They can appreciate the eternity of an instant of delight. They can derive a lifetime of pleasure from a moment of bliss. Best of all, they can give completely of themselves without asking for anything in return!

You don't have any time for nonsense, do you? Then dispense with all the impediments to your senses! Let yourself feel, experience, taste, smell, see everything you can! You are here to live!

My husband, Milton, is a marvellous lover. He makes love to me almost every night! Almost Monday, almost Tuesday, almost...

Mrs. Milton Berle

SECTION 7
SELF-HELP
Finding Safe and Healing Places

Where Do I Go for Self-Help?

Self-Hypnosis Techniques

Hypnosis is a medically approved intervention that you can do yourself. It is of great help in dealing with the physical and emotional aspects of illness, and we'd like to teach it to you.

Many people have some bizarre preconception of hypnosis as something someone else does to you. Actually, all hypnosis is self-hypnosis! Are you aware of the shoes on your feet right now? Most of us are not aware of them unless our attention is directed to them. The same thing applies to the clothes on our bodies. Most of us learn to disregard these sensations unless there's some reason why we should pay attention to them. That's a form of self-hypnosis. Thus, you're doing self-hypnosis right now, whether you know it or not! Yes, you! These lessons are learned early in life and probably began with our first pair of shoes.

Do you remember your first pair of shoes? Come on, of course you do! You were eleven months old. Your shoes were white and laced up round the ankles, and you hated them! Remember how you tried to kick them off? You even tried to untie the laces, but your hands were too clumsy and unfamiliar with the task. After a while you finally gave up and allowed your mind to turn off the sensation of the shoes on your feet, and you went back to sucking your thumb. Before long, you forgot to notice whether you had shoes on or not, you were too busy learning to walk.

If an eleven-month child can learn to turn off unnecessary sensations, you can do the same. You're doing it right now with regard to your clothing, shoes, wristwatch, etc. (No, I do not believe that you're sitting there absolutely naked reading this chapter!! If you are, you've already learned to disregard the expectations of others, which is a very important step toward health. Now, put your clothes back on and let's go to work!)

All right! All right! I'll tell how to get started! Learning to relax is the first part. That's not so hard. Here's one way. Have you ever had the experience of soaking in a hot tub at the end of a busy day when it was too much trouble to move anything at all? Good! Let yourself have that same feeling right now. Notice how comfortable and heavy your body feels — almost as if a magic paintbrush were painting back and forth over your body, erasing any tension and replacing it with a lovely pastel shade of comfort and peace. See the color of peacefulness vividly. What color is it for you? For me, it's a lovely aquamarine.

Sometimes I like to think of a beautiful tropical sunset with a fiery red sun sinking into a tranquil blue sea. For me, the sun represents the tensions I might be feeling at the moment, and the sea is the enormous reservoir of tranquillity available to extinguish those feelings. I particularly like to notice the colors as they change from red to pink and then purple, and eventually a delightfully serene blue. I also like to notice that unique stillness that occurs just at sunset when the surface of the water is like glass, the breeze is stilled, a quiet hush pervades everything, and sounds carry great distances. At those times, it's almost as if I can hear a melodious voice whispering, "RELA-A-A-A-X . . ."

By the way, how are you feeling right now? See how easy it is? Now wouldn't it be convenient if you could turn on that delightful, relaxed feeling anytime you wished? Well, you can! All you have to do is choose a signal to which your mind can respond at any time with an instant wave of relaxation. Think of this as a magic button which instantly turns on self-hypnosis. Whenever you choose to turn on this switch, it will be your signal to become totally relaxed (we call that going into trance).

My personal switch consists of making an "okay" sign with my fingertips. I do this by letting my index finger and my thumb form a circle while touching at the very tips. Whenever I do this, I feel as if I have just been magically transported to a lovely tropical island at sunset. I enjoy noticing all of the beautiful colors, the gentle movements of the palms and the waves, the fragrance of the tropical flowers, the sounds of the surf, the cool texture of the sand by the water's edge, and even the taste of a piece of tropical fruit!

I find that the moment I allow my finger and thumb to meet, I feel a sudden rush of relaxation flood through my body. I've even had occasions when, without knowing it, I was feeling tense and my finger and thumb came together automatically, with the result that I felt a sudden wave of relaxation and then noticed that my finger and thumb had come together. It's rather like an emotional thermostat that senses tension and operates on its own.

Now you try it. Let your thumb and forefinger touch.

There, did you feel anything? Of course, you felt your finger!!! I meant did you feel anything else? Did you feel a heaviness in your forearms? Or a raggedy-doll feeling in your body? If you didn't, you will. All it takes is a little practice. I suggest that you practice allowing that lovely relaxed feeling to permeate through your body once an hour throughout the day. It needn't take more than a few seconds each time. Just let your fingers come together, take a deep breath, hold it for a long delicious moment, and then let the breath out, exhaling any tension and stress with it. Feels pretty good, doesn't it?

By the way, you can do this anywhere. You can do it by yourself or while talking to someone. You can do it at home or on the job. I know of no employers who prohibit their employees from breathing on the job! As a matter of fact, it's very enjoyable to be able to remain cool and comfortable while those around you are becoming increasingly upset. It also annoys them immensely!

I like to think of my relaxation practice as rather like putting a coin into an emotional parking meter once an hour and getting two hours of comfort out of it. When practicing relaxation, or self-hypnosis, it isn't necessary to have a lengthy agenda for discussion with one's self. For example, it isn't necessary to tell yourself to relax the tightness in your chest, the tension in the back of your neck, or the butterflies in your stomach. Your mind knows how to do this just by responding to whatever cue you choose. You can use a color, a number, three deep breaths, my thumb and forefinger idea, or the simple instruction, "RELAX."

What sensation, recurrent thought, or fear would you like to get rid of first? Pain? That's the easiest of all! Have you ever had your arm or leg fall asleep? Of course, you have. Your mind already knows what that feels like and knows how to do it. Wouldn't it be nice if you could "put to sleep" the part of your body that's in pain? Well, you can!

First, practice with your hand. Which hand? I don't care which you choose. Just close your eyes and visualize your hand as if it were made of transparent material such as plastic or cellophane.

Of course, I know that you can't read these instructions with your eyes closed! Read a sentence, do what I say, and then open your eyes and read the next instruction. Or, if you prefer, allow yourself to become totally relaxed with your eyes open and then read the instructions.

Now, let's get back to visualizing your hand as if it were transparent.

First, start by giving yourself the signal to relax.

Fine! *Now visualize your hand as if you could see through all of its layers.* Notice the tiny nerves that begin in your fingertips and join other nerves further up your arm, forming a sturdier cable leading further up your arm toward the brain.

See a switchboard in your brain with a switch for each and every part of your body. Notice that over each switch is a light indicating whether the switch is on or off. You can choose whatever colors of light you prefer — white, pink, green, blue, or red.

Find the pain switch that controls the sensation in the hand you have chosen and turn the pain switch off. Notice that the light over the switch goes out, indicating that the switch is off.

Can't feel anything different? Why should you? All you did was turn off the pain switch, but naturally you left all the other switches on. Now comes the fun!

Reach out and pinch the hand whose pain switch you turned off. Feels different, doesn't it? Almost as if it were protected by a thick leather electrician's glove. Or, perhaps as if it had been soaking in ice water for a long time. You see, your mind knows how it feels to have your hand fall asleep and is perfectly capable of reproducing that sensation.

Now turn the pain switch to that hand on but turn it off in the other hand. See how simple that was? We call what you've been doing "glove anesthesia."

Now, let's learn to transfer that glove anesthesia to another part of your body. *Turn off the pain switch in the original hand.* Test it to be sure the switch is really off. It is? Good!

Now take that hand and place it on another part of your body.
Perhaps the side of your face would do for starters.

Let all the comfort transfer itself from your hand to your face.

When that has been accomplished, *let your hand drift down into your lap.* Notice that, as your hand drifts downward, the side of your face becomes more and more numb. Go ahead, it's okay to test it. How does the one side of your face feel compared with the other side? Different, isn't it?

Well, you can do the same thing with any other part of your body. All you have to do is find the pain switch that controls the sensation in that part of your body and turn it off! Simple, isn't it? And the best part is that it becomes easier to do the more you practice! What you've just been doing is self-hypnosis.

Self-hypnosis can help you in a variety of ways. We've just discussed how it can help reduce pain. Now let's talk about some other uses.

So far we've been talking about positive self-hypnosis. Negative self-hypnosis occurs when you permit someone to give you hypnotic suggestions that are not helpful. What? Who would do such a thing?? Everybody!! Let's start with the helpful soul who tells you, "This shouldn't hurt too much," just before beginning to inflict some new and hideous insult to your body. Your subconscious mind knows that what they're really saying is, "If I do this right, this should hurt like crazy!" Naturally, being a good and obedient subconscious mind, it does its very best to fulfill the expectation.

Well, how do you take care of this problem? Simple! Plan to block negative suggestions even before they are given. Just tell yourself, "If anyone says anything that is less than helpful, I simply won't be able to understand them. It will be as if they are speaking a foreign language that I don't understand." You can also tell yourself, "No matter what anyone says or does, it will only serve to make me more comfortable, relaxed, and at ease."

Let's talk about nausea associated with medications. One of the reasons that certain medications cause nausea is that everyone expects them to cause it! We've already discussed the helpful souls who tell you that all chemotherapy not only causes you to become extremely nauseated but to lose your hair and sex drive as well. Nonsense!! Some drugs do cause nausea, but most don't!

How can you use self-hypnosis to deal with the ones that do? The first thing is to block the negative suggestions that nausea is necessary for the drugs to work properly. Next, prevent any undesirable feeling from intruding on your consciousness by practicing relaxing frequently throughout the day — at least once an hour, if only for an instant. If you need to, buy yourself one of those cheap digital watches that beeps on the hour. (They'll love you in the theater and at church!)

Another useful approach is to close your eyes and remember a particularly wonderful dining experience. Perhaps at a special restaurant or at a holiday meal with relatives or a memorable meal at home. Remember how wonderfully hungry you were waiting to try all the delicious goodies spread out before you? Quick! Take an emotional snapshot of that delightfully hungry feeling and let it occur whenever you're even thinking about *thinking* about becoming nauseated. You see, you can't be hungry and nauseated at the same time.

Some people prefer to think of a switch that controls any negative feelings and then turn it off along with the light above it. An alternative approach is to visualize a house with many rooms. Notice that each room contains a different feeling. Go to the room containing the feeling you wish to eliminate and turn the light switch off! Leave the lights burning brightly in the rooms with good feelings.

As you can see, you are limited only by your imagination with regard to using your mind to alter the way your body feels. One last approach is to pass your body through a magic mirror. Leave all the good feelings in the part of your body on this side of the mirror and let all the bad feelings be on the other side of the mirror.

Well, I hope you're getting the hang of it by now. If you're interested in reading further on the subject, you might check out a copy of a paperback entitled *Self-Hypnosis* by Leslie LeCron from your local library. It was written a while ago but is still very useful, readable, and has recently been reprinted.

 Hypnosis is a wonderful way to take a mini-vacation without facing rush hour traffic.

Ronna Fay Jevne

How Do I Escape the Chaos?

Stillpoints

"I was on a small island in the South Pacific. From the northwest corner, I could view the island interior as well as the expansive and powerful Pacific. The island was an oval shape depressed in the center, as islands of volcanic origin often are. Dense tropical forest surrounded a large clear pond in the center of the island. A number of children were nearby. We seemed to be preparing a clearing for some future undefined purpose. I had walked to the crest of the island to enjoy the view during a short rest period. It seemed inevitable that we would perish in the approaching tidal wave. It was obviously futile to seek shelter. To go below the tree line would be sure death. That I could not swim seemed of little consequence. I heard the thought, 'I need a stillpoint.' It came quietly and firmly. I stood perfectly still. It felt as if time stood still. A mist surrounded me, and where a riptide or undercurrent should have been, a vacuum of safety had been created. There was a sense of total calmness. When the tidal wave had passed, the children, although bruised and distressed, were also safe. The hillside had been stripped and the island ravaged.

"I was concerned about a resort nestled on the southeast side of the island. As I neared it, I could see it had been badly damaged. The guests, however, were just arriving back from a day excursion, and a smorgasbord had been set up as best it could be to feed the group. I sought out a friend I knew to be in the group. In response to my inquiry, 'Are you all right?' she replied, 'Of course, threat is only the hell you create in your own mind.' "[1]

Have you ever felt as if time stood still? Or wished that it would stand still at a given moment? Then you have had a stillpoint. You have known that very special sense of feeling astonishingly safe in the midst of threat and turmoil. If you have not, then you can develop a stillpoint if you choose.

Why a stillpoint? Because with a stillpoint comes the ability to feel strength and calmness apart from the relentless hassles and challenges that coping and recovering from an illness often present.

Coping and recovering from a serious illness present endless problems. If you are a good problem-solver, you do well for some time. You may even be exceptional at coping with problems. However, time and symptoms can start to wear you down. Frustration, doubt, and/or fear begin to creep in. Solving everything and dealing with everything logically does not resolve everything. Not all problems and feelings are logical and, consequently, nor are all solutions. And some things escape resolution at certain points.

Stillpoints are a technique that allow you to stay calm and feel safe in the midst of threat. They are like the eye of a hurricane, providing some place safe regardless of the apparent or obvious threat. They allow you to get on with what needs to be done without blocking feelings.

A stillpoint is not a sense of being in control of everything. It is a sense of confidence that things are as predictable as possible and that they will work out as best they can. It is a state without fear and without judgment. A stillpoint is like an emotional companion. It is the oasis in a desert. A stillpoint strengthens the spirit to deal with that which may be beyond one's control. *Sometimes doing more, controlling more, trying harder is not the answer.* The more effort you put into controlling what is truly outside of your control, the more anxious, frustrated, and powerless you will feel. You need the ability to differentiate what is and what is not under your control. For the former, managing your time, communicating well, and problem-solving all will help. For the latter, a stillpoint will allow you to take charge,

[1]Excerpt from "Creating Stillpoints: Beyond a Rational Approach to Counseling Cancer Patients," by Ronna Fay Jevne, Ph.D. *Journal of Psychosocial Oncology*, Vol. 5 (3), Fall 1987. Used by permission of The Haworth Press.

not of the situation per se, but of your *response* to it. A stillpoint is difficult to describe but comforting and powerful to experience.

Having a stillpoint is not synonymous with being quiet, calm, or objective. Indeed, it actually allows you to feel all of your feelings without judgment. No energy is spent in deciding if you should or should not be feeling something. You just are who you are. You come to accept that your anger is as valuable as your tears, that confusion is the forerunner to clarity, and that discouragement often comes before feeling stronger. There is a deep sense of accepting what it means to be human — the vulnerabilities and strengths. There is a sense of trust in one's self and a sense of being connected with a source of power greater than what we are alone. Each of us may vary in terms of our thoughts as to the source of that energy. However, there seems to be a consensus that there is a power or resource beyond our rational, reasonable, problem-solving self which we can access.

In a stillpoint there is a very strong sense of being only in the present. Think about it. Fear is usually embedded in a bad memory or experience, or in anticipation of the future. At any given moment, there is no need for fear. There may be a need for action, but there is no advantage to being afraid.

In Relaxation and Mental Training classes run at our hospital for patients and families, we began to experiment with the idea of still-points. Much to my surprise, the participants seemed immediately to identify with the idea. They enjoyed sharing their sense of stillpoint with each other. Many began to work on increasing their capacity to sustain a stillpoint.

Having basic self-hypnosis skills can make it easier to get a sense of your stillpoint. Why not relax right now? Ask yourself, given what understanding you now have of a stillpoint, would you describe your experience of it as:

- *a feeling?* Perhaps being held in the arms of someone who unconditionally loves you? Floating quietly on a cloud? Caressing clay as you create something?

- *an image?* A spectacular view? A gentle morning? A particular look in someone's eyes? (I often use the gentleness in the eyes of my husband as he said his marriage vows.)

- *a color?* A special sunrise or sunset? A mist of color acting like a shield? A rainbow? (I recall a mother who lost her son who was an avid outdoorsman. As his ashes were spread in the mountain, a brilliant rainbow broke through the clouds. On every occasion following that day when she saw a rainbow, she reexperienced the sense of joy and tenderness of that moment.)

- *a sound?* Children's laughter? The tide lapping at the beach? A symphony? Silence in a forest?

- *a smell?* A fresh rose garden? Cinnamon buns fresh from mom's oven? The freshness at a mountain stream?

- *a season?* The regeneration of spring? The quiet of fall? The power of a winter blizzard or a summer downpour?

- *a person you know?* The grandpa who was always there for you? The sister you treasure? The friend you know you can count on?

- *a story?* A favorite parable? A family classic? An inspiring quote?

- *a ritual?* Communion prayer? Meditation? Eating together with loved ones? Singing together?

- *a combination of these?*

A stillpoint is that deep quiet and okayness that you feel when you know that things are the best they can be. It does not mean that the situation is necessarily the way that you want it. It means *the situation and you are the best that they can be under the circumstances.* We talked about the difficulty and importance of being able to let go of being in control of everything and the need to trust. A stillpoint helps.

Can you recall a time when you felt a greater sense of being "still on the inside" than you do now? To what did you attribute that sense of stillness? What would be necessary for you to have that sense of stillness again now? Your logical side might answer, "I'd need to be well!" Given that you may not be well in the next few days, are you willing to forego any sense of calmness or inner peace? Try again. What would be necessary for you to have more stillness, less agitation, less worry? How are you blocking yourself from the potential for a still-point? We're not talking about what you can do to *fix* the situation; we're talking about your inner state, your spirit. It must be something within *your* control. It's not easy to *stop doing* and *start being*. If you have had a deep sense of spiritual awareness throughout your life, you will already have a foundation for a stillpoint. For those of you who may have been disconnected from the spiritual side of yourself for many years, you will welcome the sense of calm and okayness that comes with the experience.

Remember, this is a part of you that does not operate on logic. Even at this moment, you may be struggling to accept the validity of the idea of stillpoints. Look around in your life. There are probably a number of other things present in your life that are not based on logic. Do you love someone? Try to explain that from the view of reason!

Perhaps an example will help.

Jane was a young mother dedicated to her family. John, her eldest child, was seriously ill with a childhood disease. She and her husband were very capable, caring people whose marriage was straining under the pressure. They were both used to being able to control matters in their lives. Jane had done everything within her power. She had changed the family diet, read avidly, and been a companion to her son throughout the illness, as had her husband. There was no more to control or do. She was exhausted and worried constantly.

Jane reported that any sense of stillpoint she had was associated with being in the wilderness and the sense of being connected to a greater power, even though she was not religious. She had, however, begun a ritual of beginning each day with lying a few moments in bed, asking God (whom she hoped existed) to ensure her son would not die. She felt, though, that this was not helping.

Rather than going over and over the things that would help her son live, I asked, "If you had any sense of what is blocking you from having a sense of calmness and strength, what would it be?"

Tears came to her eyes as quickly as she answered, "Fear." She was deeply afraid that John would die and that "things" would fall apart.

Jane decided that her image of safety would not be tied only to the survival of her son but that her family would be safe if she had the strength and calmness to deal with whatever they had to face.

"What would need to happen for you to feel that sense of safety?" I asked Jane.

"I would have to let go of being afraid and would have to let go of trying to control everything," she responded.

Jane chose not to stop asking for her son's recovery, but to add a request for the strength and peace to cope with this challenging time. She repeated her request several times during each day.

John did die. His last hours were at home in the security of his own room and his parents' love. Jane reported with amazement that the last hours were precious and without fear. "Things" did not fall apart.

A stillpoint is a phenomenon that escapes adequate description with words. It is an experience. It is an idea that is simultaneously simple and complex. In this way it is like a form of Japanese poetry called "haiku" which casts into seventeen syllables some of the highest feelings of which human beings are capable. The shortness of the haiku has nothing to do with the significance of the content. Suzuki says this of brevity:

> "At the supreme moment of life and death, we just utter a cry or take to action, we never argue, we never give ourselves up to a lengthy talk. Feelings refuse to be conceptually dealt with. A haiku is not the product of intellection."

Neither is stillpoint. Perhaps these haiku will give you a start if you are out of touch with your stillpoint:

> "Thinking comfortable
> thoughts
> with a friend in silence
> in the cool evening."

> "The leaves never know
> which leaf
> will be the first to fall . . .
> Does the wind know?"

 In the middle of winter I at last discovered that there was in me an invincible summer.

Albert Camus

SECTION 8

ENDINGS

Death and Other Tough Goodbyes

Death Isn't Catching, Just Inevitable!

Anticipatory Grieving

This is a book written for the living, so why even talk about dying? Easy! In order to devote all of our energies to living, it's necessary to resolve our fears about dying. In other words, if we can handle the idea of dying, we can handle living! At some level each of us has to come to terms with the fact that the ratio of births to deaths is one to one. One problem about death is that we don't know when or under what circumstances we will die. As a consequence, we sense a lack of control relative to death.

This is not always the case.

> Three sailors were captured during wartime attempting to sabotage one of their opponent's ships. They were sentenced to be shot sequentially by a firing squad. The first man stood bravely in front a sea wall and, facing the firing squad, refused a blindfold. Just as the soldiers had him in their sights, he yelled, "Earthquake!" This was sufficient to distract the soldiers, and he raced off into the side streets for his getaway.
>
> The second chap, no intellectual slouch, also refused a blindfold and at just the exact moment yelled, "Tidal wave!" Again, the distraction was sufficient to allow his escape among a blaze of bullets as he leapt over the sea wall.
>
> The third man confidently also refused a blindfold. He awaited the precise moment to create a distraction and then yelled, "Fire!"

Death is an unknown and unknowns are frightening, and so it is with death. Very few of us have died before and been able to be here to share the experience. What is the best way to deal with fear of the unknown? Make it less unknown.

Do you remember the first time you went to school and how apprehensive you felt because it was a strange and new experience? Perhaps your mother even took you to the bus stop or to the school itself. (Come on, confess! Mine did, too!) After a very short while, you wouldn't dream of having anyone accompany you. It would have been too humiliating! You had become familiar with the experience, and the fear had vanished.

We can't assure you that you can become totally comfortable with the death experience, but we can help you have some insight into how it feels. We have used imagery to allow patients to project forward in time and thus gain insight into the death experience, which all of us will share. Without exception, this has been a comforting rather than a disturbing experience. Would you like to try?

Take a moment, find a comfortable and quiet spot, and let your mind go forward in time to a point when your death is imminent.

Where are you and what's happening?

Notice that you're not alone. Who's there with you? It's nice to know that they care enough to be with you. Perhaps you can convey to them that there's nothing wrong with helping someone to die in the same caring way that it's nice to help someone to be born. It's a lot different from *causing* someone to die!

Keep on visualizing the scene. Have you died yet? If not, I'll wait. . . If you have, what did it feel like? Like a transition from one state into another? Almost like going to sleep and waking in a different place? What kind of place is it? Your image may be different from mine, but I'm sure that it's tranquil, secure, and includes a sense of being welcomed and belonging.

Can you see your former body? How does it look? Do you think it knows you're gone yet? How do your friends and relatives act? What do they say? Of course they're sad, but don't they know that you didn't take all your love with you when you left? Those feelings, moments, and experiences were a permanent gift that can never be taken away! And what's even better is that you have an identical and original copy of those feelings to take with you as well!

Take a moment and let time progress a little further. How are you remembered? Did you prepare your loved ones well for your absence? Do they think of you often? Of course they do! It was a good idea to make those audio- or video-tapes for them to have for special occasions. That way you're always with them at times of joy as well as special times like weddings and graduations. If you're not too handy with electronic gismos, maybe you left a letter or a card. Think of how delighted your future grandchildren will be to know that you prepared special messages for them before they were even going to be born!

It's also nice to know that you won't be very far away, anyway. Many religions believe that as long as you remain alive in the memory of anyone still living, then you aren't dead at all. It's nice to know that love comes in its own indestructible package that lasts forever and can never be depleted, only added to!

Well, how do you feel about dying so far? Not too bad is it? Besides, who's to say that you can't come back? If you do, let me know — I'd love to hear from you!

Now that you're experienced in dying, let's talk about the sadness most of us feel when we think about our own or someone else's death. It may be somewhat similar to the feeling we have after watching a lovely sunset, finishing a good book, or reflecting on a first romance, only stronger. Like all difficult-to-describe times, we recognize that life is a lovely experience, but we know it cannot go on forever.

Grieving is perfectly natural and helpful. It helps us adjust to the state of affairs as they really are. It's natural to grieve over our own death, realizing that things won't be the same as they were in the past. It is important to remember that it is a delight to have been able to experience life in the first place and to realize that our experiences will always be with us and with those with whom we shared them!

It's also natural to regret not being able to do and feel things. There is a sense of sadness at the awareness of lost opportunities, relationships that will never happen, goals that won't quite be achieved, or dreams that will have to be set aside. We want it all. The final letting go of what has *not* been is difficult. This may be a time that you want to actively grieve a loss of what could not be.

On the other hand, it's not good to be constantly grieving to the extent that it compromises enjoying life as we now have it. There are some individuals who are professional mourners. They serve a purpose.

They remind us to be grateful for the current experience that we may never have again, but they can be a real drag at a party.

Each of us will have to face our own death in our own way. Yet no one says you have to face death alone. Your faith will be with you — and this can be faith in God, in yourself, or both. Each of us has to develop an approach to death that is most appropriate for ourselves.

Preparing for something allows us to make choices about how we wish to deal with life. However, preparing for death does not mean that we wish it to occur! All of us have spare tires in our cars, but few of us go around trying to get a flat tire in order to be able to use the spare! The same thing applies to death!

If you do have to face unfortunate timing for the end of life, at least get what you want from the time you have. Live life to the fullest, take every reasonable — and even some unreasonable — risks. Compress a lifetime of living into every instant of time. And, above all, waste no time on nonsense!

Each blade of grass, each flower in the field lays down its life in its time as beautifully as it took it up.

Henry David Thoreau

The Dog Ate My Cookie

Dealing with Grief

The family had finished supper, but the little boy was still dutifully eating all of his carrots and peas which his mother had insisted he finish before he was allowed to eat the large frosted cookie that she had baked especially for him. As instructed, he left the table to wash his hands before eating dessert. Upon his return, he found his former best friend looking very self-satisfied while licking the last few crumbs off his nose and paws. "Mommy!" the boy sobbed, "the dog ate my cookie!"

A lovely little angel complete with wings and halo rang the doorbell on Halloween eve. She looked all of five years old and had long blond hair and a missing front tooth. After sweetly announcing, "Trick or treat!" she held out her pillow case containing her accumulated loot, eagerly anticipating even more goodies. An apple was dropped into the pillow case and a crunching sound was heard as it hit the bottom. The sweet little angel looked down into the pillow case, then up with narrowed eyes and chin set forward, while saying, "You broke my *#@☆*! potato chips."

Each child was acknowledging grief — the natural and universal expression of loss. Many life transitions have inherent in them a component of loss. When we are born, we lose the security of the womb. On our first day of school we lose the boundaries of home and some of our freedom.

Can you recall the first loss of a loved object? Was it your teddy? A pet? A grandparent?

You have already adjusted to the loss of many things. Loss begins with birth and ends with death and never stops in between. Death is simply the final loss as we know it. It may not be the greatest loss.

You likely have already lost your status as a child, an unattached person, a student, a dependent. But notice! You have *gained* the status of an adult, partner, employable person, responsible person.

You may have had experiences where you felt you lost your innocence, your confidence, your vibrancy, or your trust in people. You can lose your sense of responsibility, your sense of community, your sense of humor, or your common sense. You can lose your money, your job, your loved ones, or your health. You can experience loss suddenly or gradually. The loss may be painful or a blessing. You may be prepared or surprised. You can be accepting or angry or numbed. You may be loud about it or keep it very much to yourself.

How you react will be influenced by *what* you lost. How important was it to you? How did the loss occur? What was your relationship with the lost object, function, or person? What is your own personality like, and the society or family in which you live? In other words, loss is a personal and individual matter. No two people will react in exactly the same way.

Loss may be accompanied by a variety of signs of grief. Your usual routine may feel less satisfying. Motivation and concentration will probably be down. You may not feel like finishing things. You may start a letter and not remember to whom you are writing. Your appetite and sleep patterns may change. You may not want to see people. Ironically, you may also have a sense of needing people. General fatigue, short temperedness, and a lack of interest are signals that you are dealing with a loss. You may feel a hollow spot in your stomach, tightness in your throat, and even breathless.

You already know there are numerous losses involved in adjusting to an illness. Not facing those losses can have dire consequences. Doris, for example, was an attractive beautician who could not tolerate even the *thought* of losing her hair with chemotherapy. Granted, her hair did look lovely at her funeral.

"Grief work" is the expression used to describe the task of coming to terms with a loss. Gradually it is important to:

- Accept the reality of the loss.

- Acknowledge the feelings that accompany your loss.

- Say goodbye to one phase of life.

- Say hello to another phase of life.

Grieving is hard work. It zaps your energy. Oh, you may bury yourself in work for a while, or have the energy to rage, but, basically, grieving temporarily depletes you of joy and optimism.

Healing takes time. When a physical injury occurs, no amount of wishing can make it heal faster. An acutely painful period of time is followed by a less excruciating period. A time of convalescence and rehabilitation are likely required before full use of the injured area is regained. However, if you ignore the injury, allow it to become infected, or demand too much of the injured area, normal healing will be jeopardized. Your non-physical self is similar.

You can prolong the recovery process if you blame yourself, deny that you are like anyone else, believe that you will not be affected, get stuck in your anger or your despair, or punish yourself or others whom love you.

You can help yourself if you:

- Believe the loss has happened.

- Be realistic about whether or not it can be reversed. (Children up to about the age of nine believe death can be reversed.)

- Understand how grief heals.[1]

- Admit to yourself how you are feeling.

- Talk and share with someone who cares.

- Make fewer demands on yourself.

- Do your best to keep on doing things and seeing people.

[1]There are many practical and helpful books available. We're particularly fond of *How to Survive the Loss of a Love* by Melba Colgrove. (See the Bibliography for complete reference.) It is helpful for all kinds of losses.

- Take good physical and emotional care of yourself through the grieving process.

Take a moment to take stock.

- What are the losses you are dealing with?

- How are you dealing with them?

- Have you even admitted you are hurting?

- Does it feel as if your grief is healing?

- Is there anything you need to do to keep the healing process happening?

There are no losses without the possibility for gains. But to benefit from a loss, we must do more than passively endure loss. A loss is an emotional injury. It wounds our trust, our stability, our energy, our motivation, perhaps even our view of the world.

If you broke your arm, in all likelihood it would be casted to protect it so the healing process could begin. However, your arm wouldn't recover its strength if you never exercised it. In the first part of rehabilitation, it probably would feel weak and perhaps even painful. Similarly, with loss. At first it is appropriate to protect one's self, but eventually you have to start doing things. It may seem painful to engage in life again, but the emotional cast must come off. And it may be difficult. Very difficult, depending on the loss. At first, you can likely think of no possible gain, but as time heals and competence in living returns, you may acquire a sensitivity, wisdom, and strength that was not previously obvious. It doesn't mean you necessarily stop hurting or missing the person, but you are more able to live because they were part of your world.

For example, if you have lost someone whom you used to consult for advice and support, notice that they are still there for you. You can ask yourself, "How would _____ have handled this?" Their skill will now have become your skill and strength.

Healing life's hurts has been subject matter for many a great author, poet, and philosopher. To adjust to the relentlessness of loss in our lives is to accept the invitation to understand fully what it means to be human. There can be no sense of loss without a sense of attachment, and there are no meaningless attachments!

Life is a series of losses and gains. The challenge is in learning which is which.

Ronna Fay Jevne

Handle with Care, Then Pass It On

Caring for Loved Ones

You can never repay the people in your life for all the love and kindnesses they have shown you in the past. Think about all your relatives, friends, teachers, and even strangers who have shared their love with you throughout your lifetime. Some of them may even be dead now, but their kindness lives on in your memory. Love is that way — it never dies! Once generated, love remains forever. It may lie waiting, dormant in a letter or a painting, waiting for another individual to discover it and, by so doing, revive it once again.

The way to repay people for having shared their love with you is to pass that love on to someone else! There can never be too much love in the world, and each time you generate a little more, it adds to the supply available for all of us. You don't have to do anything extremely complex in order to generate love. It can happen by sharing a smile with a stranger, petting a dog, or even writing a book.

This book is our way of sharing our love with you. We can never repay all the wonderful people who have helped and inspired us throughout the years, but we can try to help others and ask them to pass it on!

You can do the same thing. If you learn something useful from this book, pass it on! If you make a discovery that helps you be more comfortable or happier, pass it on! If someone gives you a smile, pass it on! And if someone shares their love with you, pass it on! Don't expect to receive any reward other than the good feeling that comes from sharing something you treasure with another. It's interesting, isn't it, how even the most beautiful sunset is lovelier when there is someone there to share it with you. Share the warmth of your love with others, and you will have the same contented, peaceful feeling. AND IT WILL LAST FOREVER!

Who needs to be told that you love them? Everyone! No one else can do it for you. This is one thing you have to do for yourself. Get started right away! We'll wait!

There are some specific ways you can tell people that you love them and ensure that the love will be available for them whenever they need it. Write it down or tape record it. Leave messages that your loved ones can consult at appropriate times. A legacy of love only becomes more valuable with the passage of time! Love can be shared in many ways.

One gift that we give to each other is the memories we share. The child of a sick mother can be left with the memory of a bedridden, depressed mother or the memory of long hours snuggled next to a loving mother who listened to the child read for hours at a time. An ill man can leave behind the memory of remorse over not having achieved financial success, or the memory that he faced circumstances bravely and set an example for others to follow.

Will the memories you leave be of comfort to those you love? In their minds will they hear the sound of your laughter and your words of encouragement? Will they recall your strength and humanity, as well as your tenderness and concern? Will they be better equipped to share with others for having shared in your life? Will they be better equipped for the challenges in their lives because of having participated in yours?

Planning ahead for the well-being of those you care for demonstrates your love. Helping someone you love deal with the pain or fear of losing you is a very precious gift. Writing a will or prearranging a funeral is another way of showing them how much you care. Facilitating communication is another.

Talk to people and resolve any grievances that may exist. Plan ahead and avoid any future grievances. If you have certain possessions that you would like certain persons to have, tell them now or give them the items now.

Or go ahead and get well, so that you can continue to share love and happiness for many years to come. Fight for all you are worth to recover, but at the same time realize that what makes some things precious is their rarity and the fact that they do not last forever. Roses don't always grow in the winter, but they will always be there in your memory just as fresh and as fragrant as ever! Share the roses of your memory with others!

If you feel you are all alone and without anyone to depend on, you can enrich your life by setting an example for all of us. You can teach us how to deal with adversity and how to make a contribution which will benefit all.

During illness you are taken out of the mainstream of life. After the initial crises and support, people return to their jobs and daily commitments. Your world may get smaller and smaller. You may need to make a conscious commitment to remember you are a valuable, capable, lovable person who is presently ill. Illness doesn't make you worthless, inadequate, or unlovable. In our age of hurry and overcommitment, it's easy to fall prey to feelings of being abandoned during illness.

Ironically, you will be much less likely to be alone if you can maintain your self-worth. This is not the same as being selfish. It is recognizing the worth of your *self*. We know it isn't easy.

They say that former schoolteachers are never lonely in their old age because they have developed the ability to communicate and make friends with people younger than themselves. They have developed a sense of self-worth that transcends age barriers.

Not infrequently, a person whose entire life seems to have been devoted to selfish interests will change in the face of serious illness and develop a capacity to share love and warmth. They find that being forced to *really* look at what is truly important enables them to grow both spiritually and emotionally. How about you?

We accept that there is no right way to live and no right way to die. There is only the way that each of us can do it at the time. We accept that your way may not be our way, but we also accept that we can learn from each other, and that if we all do what we can, all of our suffering will be a little less. We can share understanding, but in all probability no one can understand what you are going through. We can say, however, that we respect the fact that you're doing the best you can.

Accept the inevitable with good humor and grace. It's not up to us to understand why some things happen and others don't. It is up to us to be grateful for all the gifts which we do receive.

The story is told about the minister in Tennessee
who went for a walk in the woods on a sunny day. He
was walking along, lost in his thoughts, until he heard a

crashing noise off to the side. He looked over and saw an enormous black bear running directly at him about three hundred yards away.

He then did what any self-respecting minister would do. He put his hands together, closed his eyes, and prayed, "Dear Lord, please help me in my hour of need!" He then quickly opened his eyes and saw that the bear was now only two hundred yards away!

The minister then prayed once again, "Dear Lord, I have been a good and faithful servant of yours all these years. Please come to my aid!" He opened his eyes again and saw that the bear was only one hundred yards away.

He knew this was his last chance as he prayed, "Dear Lord, I have much of your work still unfinished, but if you wish to call me to you, Thy will be done!"

He opened his eyes and discovered the bear sitting three feet away with the most benevolent smile on its face. The minister breathed a great sigh of relief and said, "THANK GOD!"

At which point the bear put his paws together, looked up and said, "For what I am about to receive, may I be truly grateful!"

No matter what we have received, we all have reason to be truly grateful! Whatever you have, *pass it on*.

 Love is the leading cause of life.

Ashleigh Brilliant

SECTION 9

CONCLUSION

What's the Next Step?

The New Graduate

Tools and Strategies

Congratulations! You've just completed the short course in how to survive. Now it's up to you to practice using your new tools. If we've done our job well, by now you should be familiar with your tool box.

Remember the basics. These are the major tools:

- your healthcare team
- your support system
- your attitude
- access to information
- communication skills
- your inner resources
- faith

Let's check inside. Yes, there's:

- the importance of communicating
- the naturalness of feeling
- the uniqueness of each person
- the value of managing your own life
- your potential to overcome adversity

The strategies to use the tools are endless, limited only by your creativity and willingness to try them. Why not keep a list nearby to help during those times you are stuck or just feeling adventuresome?

- journal writing
- self-hypnosis
- imagery
- humor
- art
- music
- reading
- communicating more effectively
- handling feelings more effectively
- getting more assertive
- distracting yourself
- taking one problem at a time
- having goals
- setting priorities
- sharing yourself

You're still alive. You've read this book. You're interested in action. You have courage to face the challenges. Go for it.

It has been fun writing to you. How about writing to us? One of our greatest pleasures is working with and hearing from people who have been told they would not survive. Tell us what you have done to get over the tough spots. Tell us your anecdotes, skills, or frustrations. You heard us out. Now it's your turn to be heard. Either or both of us would love to hear from you. If you would like a response from us, please enclose a self-addressed, stamped envelope, and we'll be pleased to respond.

Ronna Fay Jevne
6-102 Education North
Dept. of Educational Psychology
University of Alberta
Edmonton, Alberta, CANADA
T6G 2G5

Alexander Levitan
500 Osborne Road, Box 115
Fridley, Minnesota 55432

 Fear and freedom are mutually exclusive.

Eric Hoffer

Love Means Living On

Survival Tactics for Loved Ones

*STOP! This chapter is not for you, if you are the person
with the life-threatening illness. It is for those who care
about and for you. We have some advice for them, too.*

Now that we're alone, let's talk about some of the things that you've
been thinking and feeling. Yup! It's perfectly normal to be angry. Who
wouldn't be? You didn't do anything to deserve this illness and neither
did the person you care about. But it happened anyway. So, what can
you do?

You can choose to remain angry and thereby make everything you
have to do become a burden. Or, you can accept what has happened
as nobody's fault and carry on. If it is somebody's fault, how long do
you plan on continuing to blame them? Has blaming someone been
productive or helpful to you? Of course not! Nobody says you have
to like being stuck in this situation, but don't make it any tougher on
yourself than it has to be!

Whenever you hold on to anger, you're just surrendering control
to the situation. It's as if you just handed over your remote control
device to someone and said, "Here, play with this and make me
miserable."

So, what can you do? Press the erase button, eliminate the anger,
and start to feel good again! (If you want further suggestions, you might
want to read the chapter entitled "Go Jump in a Lake," page 132. For
that matter, you might want to read the whole book!)

Sure, all this sounds easy for us to say! But you need to know that
we've been there, too! Both of us have had serious health problems

which have at times made our lives pretty difficult. We've been angry, frustrated, depressed, and pretty darn miserable, but we've made it through . . . so far. Nope, we don't want your sympathy, just your acceptance that our knowledge is not only from a textbook or as professionals.

Of course it's unfair that all of your energy and most of your financial resources are being directed at only one person to the exclusion of everyone else. But would you really have it any other way? That's what love is all about!

Remember, if you were the one who was ill, they would be helping you.

And who says you can't help yourself? You have every right to take some time away just for yourself. That's not being selfish — that's just being smart! You wouldn't drive your car indefinitely without changing the oil, would you? Well, it's the same with your body and your mind.

Arrange to have somebody cover for you — at least one night or, even better, a weekend, and several afternoons as well. Get out and do whatever most appeals to you for relaxation. After all, if you don't take care of yourself, there's no way you can take care of anyone else! All that will happen is that there will be two patients in the family instead of one.

If you're the only one available to give the care, contact a visiting nursing organization to see what services they can provide to give you a little respite from your efforts. In some cases it may be necessary to place the person you love in a hospice unit or a nursing home so that you can get away for the weekend. Again, that isn't selfish, that's smart! Doing it the first time is the hardest.

You may also be surprised to find out that your loved one may be eligible for a variety of services at no cost. In the United States, The Cancer Society frequently provides hospital beds, commodes, and a variety of such equipment at no cost. Similarly, once a patient is certified for hospice care under Medicare, they no longer have to pay for medications, hospital, nursing, or doctor's care. The program picks up all these bills.

Because Canadians share the cost of medical services through a national healthcare scheme, most medical bills are paid through the government program. Additional services are available through private medical insurance, and self-help organizations, such as the Canadian

Cancer Society, have Patient Services Divisions to assist with special needs.

AIDS patients have a tougher time. Frequently they exhaust their medical benefits and personal resources and have to look to public assistance for help. Fortunately, many enlightened communities, such as San Francisco, have developed and funded numerous community involvement programs for exactly this situation. More communities are learning to develop these types of programs as well.

Similarly, there are a great many programs that provide assistance to caregivers and families of seriously ill patients. Find out about them! Call the local home care agency and ask what they can do. Call your city, county, state, or province welfare agency and see if you or your loved one are eligible for any benefits. Call the social service department in your local hospital and have them tell you what programs are available in your community which could be of benefit to you or the person you're caring for. Remember, this is not charity; this is what you are entitled to receive! It is no different than social security, retirement benefits, or any other program to which you or your family member are entitled.

Leaves of absence from work may also be appropriate on occasion. Talk to your employer if this would fit your needs. You'll also find that there are programs for arranging for a family member to be brought home from the military if it is deemed necessary. Similarly, compassionate discharges can be arranged when appropriate.

By the way, you'll also find out that seriously ill persons like to have some time to themselves. It gets tiring to have even the most well-meaning individual hovering around all the time. As you've no doubt discovered, if the person you're caring for needs something, you'll be asked for it.

Now, let's talk about some of the other thoughts or feelings you've been having. Yes, it's perfectly normal to wish that it were all over, even if that means that the person you're caring for would be dead. You're not a terrible person for wishing that your mother, brother, child, or lover were dead under these circumstances. Many people have said, "It's more comfortable for me to think of him/her as dead rather than deal with the uncertainty!"

We recommend you attend a support meeting for those who care for seriously ill patients where you can share some of these taboo thoughts and find out that we all have them! Certain hospitals and care organizations have weekend retreats for patients and those who care for them to facilitate these discussions. See if any are going on in your area.

Now, let's talk about the organization. What? You didn't know you were a member of one? Of course you are! The trick is to organize it so that it functions optimally. Children, parents, friends, lovers, and other members of an extended family can be of enormous help if properly given the opportunity to be so. There's no reason why you have to do everything yourself!

Begin by calling an organizational meeting. If necessary, post notices so that those members who are normally either out or at home in coma (e.g., teenagers) are aware of the meeting and able to attend. Start by drawing up a list of duties normally performed by the patient. Then distribute these responsibilities among the remaining members. Make sure everyone clearly understands what they are responsible for doing.

Even very young children can sweep the floor, sort the laundry, and take out the garbage. Basically, all of the chores can be divided up, with the understanding that if anyone feels overloaded or wishes to exchange responsibilities, they may reconvene the council to discuss the matter. In any event, it is a good idea to have a formal meeting once a week to discuss matters of common interest, including feelings.

Don't be afraid to involve the patient in any of these discussions, if they wish to be. You don't want them feeling that things are being done behind their back or that they are letting you down. Let them do whatever they feel like doing and, if it's too much, arrange for someone else to take over. At certain times it may be appropriate for a temporary take-over by another family member or helper; at other times, it may be a more permanent take-over of responsibility. The patient should be reassured when a temporary change is made that they may resume a particular responsibility whenever they are able. It's important for ill people to feel needed and to know that they still have something important to contribute to the family. Remember: The most important responsibility of the ill person is to get well or to be comfortable, depending on the stage of their illness.

Don't be afraid to be realistic. Patients can take the truth. What they can't take is someone trying to deceive them. When appropriate, it's okay to give a patient permission to stop trying. Sometimes patients feel they have to hang on because it is what their loved ones expect.

Giving them permission to let go can be a great kindness and relief to them.

Don't be afraid to discuss anything with an ill person. This can include where they want to be buried, what type of funeral service they might wish to have, and what it feels like to die. Obviously, timing is an issue, but don't make it an excuse to avoid the real issues. Also discuss the matter of heroic measures to sustain life and whether they wish to donate any organs after death.

Basically, discuss everything! One of the more common regrets that many people have is that they were unable to discuss certain matters with loved ones before they died. Don't let that happen to you!

Enough of the DON'Ts! DO cherish every moment with your loved one. DO get rid of retained anger. DO communicate effectively with your loved on and those caring for him or her. After all, you also have "No Time for Nonsense."

The best thing to hold onto in this world is each other.

Greene's Rule from 1001 Logical Laws

Don't Spit in the Soup

Professionals' Use of the Book

> *Here is your big opportunity. Your doctors/caretakers may be giving you lots of advice. Now you can share some of your knowledge with them. This chapter will help them understand some of the things you have been learning in this book. Pass it on!*

We wrote this book to help seriously ill patients, their families, friends, and you, the dedicated people who care for them. We've tried to distill many years of experience and patient contact into this book. Along the way we've also made more than our share of mistakes, and we hope we have profited from them. We have no data to suggest that the strategies introduced in this book will materially increase the length of survival of patients, but we do have good support for the fact that the quality of survival will be much improved. We know that you won't agree with everything we say, but that's fine. All we ask is that you hear us out and then make up your own mind.

One of the legitimate concerns of any healthcare practitioner, when referring a patient for help, centers around the qualifications of the party to whom the patient is being referred. It might help you to know that Ronna Fay Jevne is a chartered psychologist with a Ph.D. in counseling psychology and is currently an Associate Professor of Educational Psychology at the University of Alberta in Edmonton, Alberta, Canada. Before joining the University, she was the senior psychologist at the Cross Cancer Hospital in Edmonton.

Alexander Levitan is an M.D. who is Board-Certified in Medical Oncology, Internal Medicine, and Medical Hypnosis. He has been a practicing oncologist for twenty years and teaches at the University of Minnesota, as well as at the Illinois School of Professional Psychology.

Feel free to disagree with us. Heavens knows, we disagree with each other. But, let's agree to disagree without harming anyone, especially not the patients. You may feel that some of the things we suggest for patients will have no ultimate effect on their disease and survival, but as long as you don't feel that the suggestions will do any harm, please allow the patients to decide for themselves.

At this point we hope that you are questioning what you, as a professional, might do to further help your patients in their quest to regain good health.

One of the simplest things you could do is to make this book available, perhaps in your waiting room, for your patients, their families, and friends. It is written so that they can pick it up and read a different chapter whenever they wish.

As you know, patients hear only part of what they are told and tend to make the most pessimistic interpretation of any ambiguities which they may hear. At one time, this probably had a survival advantage for primitive people who would have been foolish not to interpret a sound outside the cave as a saber tooth tiger looking for lunch, rather than an eager partner interested in mating.

In addition to their natural propensity for pessimistic interpretation, patients get enough bad news. This is particularly true these days when there is so much emphasis on informed consent and prevention of litigation. We're sure you already do this, but if at all possible, please leave a candle of hope flickering in the window for seriously ill patients. Tell the patients the truth, but leave room for optimism if at all possible.

Most of us have read about or seen cases of spontaneous remission of very advanced, usually fatal, diseases. Few of us, if any, know how or why these remissions occur. Who is to say that your patient might not be one of these cases? If no room is left for hope, we feel that this likelihood, although rare under the best of circumstances, will be even less likely to occur.

If you've seen even one case of advanced pancreatic cancer who has lived longer than five years, we're sure all your current patients with pancreatic cancer would like to hear about it. If you'd like to read more about this subject of remissions, we suggest you look at "A Compilation of 400 Cases of Spontaneous Remissions from Cancer" by Pepper and Pelletier. (See Bibliography.)

This whole business of telling the truth, while leaving room for optimism, brings up the subject of communication. It is important to remember that we communicate in more ways than merely speaking and writing. A smile, a frown, a shrug, and a handshake all communicate our true thoughts and feelings to our patients. We suggest that you become aware of *how*, as well as *what*, you communicate. Perhaps you have had the experience of standing out of earshot, watching one of your colleagues talk to a patient's family and you could tell what type of news was being conveyed.

You can make a significant contribution to the longevity of your patients by the way you tell them things, not only verbally but through your expression, mannerisms, and enthusiasm. Be realistic but positive in your communications with patients. Tell the truth but remember to leave a little window of hope open somewhere.

Help your patients set realistic goals. Cure may not be possible but making it to a graduation next spring might be. Help give them a reason to live, not die. Their health may be compromised, but they are still valuable.

We've found that one of the most important predictors for long term survival is the patient's attitude toward living. Become familiar with the burgeoning new field of psychoneuro-immunology. There is finally good scientific data to support the interrelationship of the mind and the immune system. A recent scientific article[1] has begun to define how the mind influences the immune system. With any luck, we may be able to apply this learning to treatment of specific diseases, such as AIDS and cancer, once we learn how to consistently manipulate the mind-body interaction.

Please help us to improve patients' attitudes. Help us by giving your patients a reason to continue living, not dying as many others may expect of them. Share your humanity with them. Show them that they still have something significant to contribute to the lives of others.

At the same time, get comfortable with your own attitudes toward death and dying. Perhaps the chapter we've written on death ("Death Isn't Catching, Just Inevitable," page 182) would be of help to you. Similarly, if you've been able to figure out a way to avoid dying, please write and tell us how. We'd love to hear from you.

---

[1]Lotz, M., Vaughan, J.H, Carson, D.A., Lotz. (1988). Effect of Neuropeptides on Production of Inflammatory Cytokines of Human Monocytes. *Science* 241: 1218-21.

In closing, we have something to say that directly concerns you. If you find yourself working sixty hours a week and getting less and less patient-oriented, perhaps you might want to read our chapter on stress — "Disarming the Alarming" (page 18). You need to think about your own health, too!

One final word: *Please, please, touch your patients whenever they visit you or you visit them!* Touch them frequently. Let them know that they are not untouchables. Neither are they disposables. Share your time with them, even if you do have a thousand and one things to do, as usual. They trust you and have given over to you the care of their most important possession: their life!

Seriously ill patients may have to die, but we hope that by all of us working together they won't have to suffer, and they will be able to die in an atmosphere of dignity and love.

Throughout this book patients are offered new recipes for living. Help us to help them but, above all, DON'T SPIT IN THE SOUP!

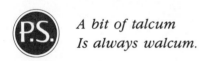

A bit of talcum
Is always walcum.

Ogden Nash

Bibliography

Alman, Brian M., with Peter T. Lambrou. 1983. *Self-Hypnosis: A Complete Manual for Health and Self-Change.* San Diego: International Health Publications.

Benjamin, Harold, and Richard Trubo. 1987. *From Victim to Victor: The Wellness Community Guide to Fighting for Recovery for Cancer Patients and Their Families.* Los Angeles: J. P. Tarcher, Inc.

Bloch, Richard, and Annette Bloch. 1986. *Cancer. . .There's Hope.* Kansas City, MO: Cancer Connection, Inc.

———. 1985. *Fighting Cancer: A Step-by-Step Guide to Helping Yourself Fight Cancer.* Kansas City, MO: Cancer Connection, Inc.

Borysenko, Joan. 1987. *Minding the Body, Mending the Mind.* Reading, MS: Addison-Wesley Publishing Company.

Brilliant, Ashleigh. 1981. *Appreciate Me Now and Avoid the Rush.* Santa Barbara, CA: Woodbridge Press.

———. 1987. *I Try to Take One Day at a Time, But Sometimes Several Days Attack Me at Once.* Santa Barbara, CA: Woodbridge Press.

Burns, George. 1984. *How to Live to Be 100 — or More.* New York: New American Library, A Signet Book.

Caprio, Frank S., and Joseph R. Berger. 1963. *Helping Yourself with Self-Hypnosis.* New York: Warner Books.

Colgrove, Melba, Harold Bloomfield, and Peter McWilliams. 1976. *How to Survive the Loss of a Love.* New York: Bantam Books.

Cousins, Norman. 1981. *Anatomy of an Illness.* New York: Bantam Books.

———. 1983. *The Healing Heart: Antidotes to Panic and Helplessness.* New York: W.W. Norton & Company.

———. 1981. *Human Options: An Autobiographical Notebook.* New York: W. W. Norton & Company.

Davis, Martha, Elizabeth Robbins Eshelman, and Matthew McKay. 1982. *The Relaxation & Stress Reduction Workbook*. Oakland, CA: New Harbinger Publications.

Dosdall, Claude, and Joanne Broatch. 1986. *My God I Thought You'd Died*. New York: Bantam Books; Toronto: Seal Books.

Dossey, Larry. 1984. *Beyond Illness: Discovering the Experience of Health*. Boulder, CO: New Science Library.

Fiore, Neil A. 1986. *The Road Back to Health: Coping with the Emotional Side of Cancer*. New York, Toronto: Bantam Books.

Gawain, Shakti. 1982. *Creative Visualization*. New York, Toronto: Bantam Books.

Glassman, Judith. 1983. *The Cancer Survivors: And How They Did It*. Garden City, NJ: Doubleday & Co., Inc.

Green, E., and A. Green. 1977. *Beyond Biofeedback*. New York: Delta.

Haley, Jay. 1984. *Ordeal Therapy: Unusual Ways to Change Behavior*. San Francisco: Jossey-Bass Inc.

Hay, Louise. 1985. *You Can Heal Your Life*. Farmingdale, NY: Coleman Publishing Inc.

Johnson, Judi, and Linda Klein. 1988. *I Can Cope: Staying Healthy with Cancer*. Minneapolis: DCI Publishing.

Kleinman, Arthur. 1988. *The Illness Narratives: Suffering, Healing & The Human Condition*. New York: Basic Books Inc., Publishers.

Kron, Errol R., and Karen Johnson. 1983. *Visualization: The Uses of Imagery in the Health Professions*. Chicago: The Dorsey Press.

Kushner, Rose. 1985. *Alternatives: New Developments in the War on Breast Cancer*. New York: Warner Books.

Lazarus, Arnold. 1977. *In the Mind's Eye: The Power of Imagery for Personal Enrichment*. New York: Guilford Press.

LeCron, Leslie M. 1964. *Self-Hypnotism: The Technique and Its Use in Daily Living*. New York: New American Library. (Reprint, New York: Prentice-Hall, 1988.)

Locke, Steven, and Douglas Colligan. 1986. *The Healer Within: The New Medicine of Mind and Body*. New York: Dutton Publishers.

Pearsall, Paul. 1987. *Superimmunity: Master Your Emotions & Improve Your Health*. New York: McGraw-Hill Book Company.

Pepper, Curtis Bill. 1984. *We, the Victors: Inspiring Stories of People Who Conquered Cancer and How They Did It*. Garden City, NJ: Doubleday & Co., Inc. (Paperback, New York: New American Library, 1985.)

Pepper, Eric, and K. Pelletier. 1976. "A Compilation of 400 Cases of Spontaneous Remission from Cancer." Circulated monograph. Sponsored by the Reynolds Foundation. (This material is reviewed in Green, E., and Green, A., *Beyond Biofeedback*.)

Peter, Laurence J., and Bill Dana. 1982. *The Laughter Prescription*. New York: Ballantine Books.

Pitzele, Sefra Kobrin. 1986. *We Are Not Alone: Learning to Live with Chronic Illness*. New York: Workman Publishing Co., Inc.

Rossi, Ernest Lawrence. 1986. *The Psychobiology of Mind-Body Healing*. New York: W. W. Norton & Company.

Rossi, Ernest Lawrence, and David B. Cheek. 1988. *Mind-Body Therapy: Methods of Ideodynamic Healing in Hypnosis*. New York: W. W. Norton & Company.

Sehnert, Keith W. 1981. *Stress—Unstress: How You Can Control Stress at Home and on the Job*. Minneapolis: Augsburg Publishing House.

Siegel, Bernie S. 1986. *Love, Medicine & Miracles*. New York: Harper & Row, Publishers, Inc. (Paperback, New York: Harper & Row, Publishers, Inc., 1988.)

Siegler, Miriam, and Humphry Osmond. 1979. *How to Cope with Illness*. New York: Collier Books.

Simonton, O. Carl, Stephanie Matthews-Simonton, and James Creighton. 1978. *Getting Well Again*. Los Angeles: J. P. Tarcher, Inc. (Paperback, New York: Bantam Books, 1980.)

Stroebel, Charles F. 1982. QR: *The Quieting Reflex*. New York: Berkley Books.

Ziebell, Beth. 1981. *Wellness: An Arthritis Reality*. Dubuque, IA, Toronto: Kendall/Hunt Publishing Company.

Ronna Fay Jevne, Ph.D.

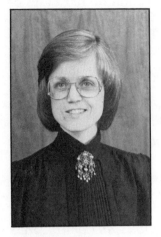

Ronna Fay Jevne, a chartered psychologist, is an Associate Professor of Educational Psychology at the University of Alberta (Edmonton, Canada) where she teaches in the masters and doctoral counseling programs. She also holds an appointment as an Associate on the Senior Scientific Staff of the Cross Cancer Institute (Edmonton) where she formerly held the position of Senior Counselling Psychologist.

Jevne's long-standing interest in chronic and life-threatening illness is reflected in her extensive experience as a practitioner, educator, consultant, and researcher in the field. Her background and specialized training is enhanced by her previous academic training in English and Philosophy.

Jevne has made numerous guest appearances throughout Canada, presenting lectures and workshops on managing the stress of illness, holistic health, loss and grieving, supportive care, and hypnotherapy.

In addition to being a founding member of the Canadian Psychosocial Oncology Association, Jevne has served her profession as an executive member of the Universities Council for the Profession of Psychology; as a reviewer for several journals, including guest editor of the *Canadian Counsellor*; and as a chairperson for the Board of Professional Examinations. Her publications include *Managing the Stress of Cancer* and *You and Stress,* as well as over thirty articles in professional journals. She is currently working on her next book, *My Spirit Can Dance*, which attempts to capture both the pain and resilience of the human spirit.

Jevne is married, has three stepchildren, two foster sons and three grandchildren, and loves photography.

Alexander Levitan, M.D.

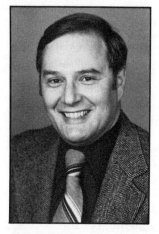

Alexander Levitan is a private practice physician who is Board-Certified in Medical Oncology, Internal Medicine, and Medical Hypnosis. He has been a practicing oncologist for twenty years and serves as a consultant in oncology and internal medicine to four Minnesota hospitals. In addition, he is a past Clinical Associate Professor at the University of Minnesota and a current associate faculty member at the Illinois School of Professional Psychology.

Levitan's unique and highly successful work in the area of clinical hypnosis has brought him much media attention. He is a recognized leader in the field of hypno-anesthesia, has made numerous television and radio appearances, and is frequently in demand as a guest speaker and workshop leader both in the United States and internationally. His contributions to medical literature and health professionals include over twenty articles and presentations on the subject of hypnosis as anesthesia, the role of touch in healing and hypnotherapy, cancer chemotherapy, and psychosocial problems of cancer patients and their families.

In addition to being President-elect of the American Society of Clinical Hypnosis, Levitan is President of the American Board of Medical Hypnosis, a member of the Board of Reviewers and Assistant Editor for the *American Journal of Clinical Hypnosis*, an Independent Investigator for the National Cancer Institute, and an honorary life member of both the Canadian and Australian Societies of Clinical Hypnosis. He has received numerous awards, including the Award of Merit for Excellence in Teaching, and the Award for Best Scientific Paper from the American Society of Clinical Hypnosis.

Levitan is married, has three daughters, and enjoys gardening and travel.

LuraMedia PUBLICATIONS

by Marjory Zoet Bankson
BRAIDED STREAMS
Esther and a Woman's Way
of Growing
(ISBN 0-931055-05-09)

SEASONS OF FRIENDSHIP
Naomi and Ruth
as a Pattern
(ISBN 0-931055-41-5)

by Alla Renee Bozarth
WOMANPRIEST
A Personal Odyssey
(ISBN 0-931055-51-2)

by Lura Jane Geiger
ASTONISH ME, YAHWEH!
Leader's Guide
(ISBN 0-931055-02-4)

by Lura Jane Geiger
and Patricia Backman
BRAIDED STREAMS
Leader's Guide
(ISBN 0-931055-09-1)

by Lura Jane Geiger, Sandy Landstedt,
Mary Geckeler, and Peggy Oury
ASTONISH ME, YAHWEH!
A Bible Workbook-Journal
(ISBN 0-931055-01-6)

by Kenneth L. Gibble
THE GROACHER FILE
A Satirical Expose of
Detours to Faith
(ISBN 0-931055-55-5)

by Ronna Fay Jevne, Ph.D.
and Alexander Levitan, M.D.
NO TIME FOR NONSENSE
Self-Help for the Seriously Ill
(ISBN 0-931055-63-6)

by Ted Loder
EAVESDROPPING ON THE ECHOES
Voices from the Old Testament
(ISBN 0-931055-42-3)

GUERRILLAS OF GRACE
Prayers for the Battle
(ISBN 0-931055-01-6)

NO ONE BUT US
Personal Reflections on
Public Sanctuary
(ISBN 0-931055-08-3)

TRACKS IN THE STRAW
Tales Spun from the Manger
(ISBN 0-931055-06-7)

by Jacqueline McMakin
with Sonya Dyer
WORKING FROM THE HEART
For Those Who Hunger for Meaning
and Satisfaction in Their Work
(ISBN 0-931055-65-2)

by Elizabeth O'Connor
SEARCH FOR SILENCE
Revised Edition
(ISBN 0-931055-07-5)

by Renita Weems
JUST A SISTER AWAY
A Womanist Vision of Women's
Relationships in the Bible
(ISBN 0-931055-52-0)

LuraMedia is a company that searches for ways to encourage personal growth, shares the excitement of creative integrity, and believes in the power of faith to change lives.

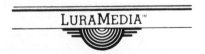
LuraMedia™